I0475585

How I Healed My Life

From Crises and Cancer
to Self-Empowerment

DAGFRID KOLAAS AND BENT MADSEN

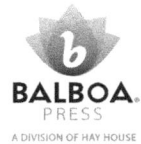

BALBOA.
PRESS
A DIVISION OF HAY HOUSE

Copyright © 2014 Dagfrid Kolaas.

All rights reserved. No part of this book may be used or reproduced by any means, graphic, electronic, or mechanical, including photocopying, recording, taping or by any information storage retrieval system without the written permission of the publisher except in the case of brief quotations embodied in critical articles and reviews.

Balboa Press books may be ordered through booksellers or by contacting:

Balboa Press
A Division of Hay House
1663 Liberty Drive
Bloomington, IN 47403
www.balboapress.com
1 (877) 407-4847

Because of the dynamic nature of the Internet, any web addresses or links contained in this book may have changed since publication and may no longer be valid. The views expressed in this work are solely those of the author and do not necessarily reflect the views of the publisher, and the publisher hereby disclaims any responsibility for them.

The author of this book does not dispense medical advice or prescribe the use of any technique as a form of treatment for physical, emotional, or medical problems without the advice of a physician, either directly or indirectly. The intent of the author is only to offer information of a general nature to help you in your quest for emotional and spiritual well-being. In the event you use any of the information in this book for yourself, which is your constitutional right, the author and the publisher assume no responsibility for your actions.

Any people depicted in stock imagery provided by Thinkstock are models, and such images are being used for illustrative purposes only. Certain stock imagery © Thinkstock.

Printed in the United States of America.

ISBN: 978-1-4525-9359-3 (sc)
ISBN: 978-1-4525-9361-6 (hc)
ISBN: 978-1-4525-9360-9 (e)

Library of Congress Control Number: 2014903739

Balboa Press rev. date: 3/7/2014

Contents

Foreword

By Rune Amundsen

Author, speaker. and ex-psychologist

Essentially, there are two ways of looking at life: either everything is meaningful or everything is meaningless. Dagfrid goes for meaning. Dagfrid goes for the idea that human beings have been given the gift by Nature—or God if you like—of being able to create their own reality.

It stands to good reason that, if we are able to make ourselves sick, we might as well use our powers to make ourselves happy and well; and what is more—and what is of utmost importance—is that the experience of sickness and health both have an intrinsic holy nature.

Dagfrid tells us a story of power—the potential power of inner knowledge and joy that had hidden itself and had lain dormant in the deepest crises of her life. Most of her life was in ruin, both in terms of social life and her faltering health. But she managed to turn it all the other way around; the crisis became a gift of renewal and inspiration for herself and the people she met along the way.

One of Dagfrid's biggest assets is courage—courage to explore ... courage to make a difference.

Her book of hope is one of those stories that "charms" and paves the way for others to find their own unique paths. She points the way to the inbuilt self-healing process of Nature and helps us ultimately to rest peacefully and joyfully in the miracle of the "aliveness" of our bodies.

Dagfrid tells a story about discovering her inner healer. Not in solitude and isolation; that is not the way of Dagfrid. Neither did Dagfrid rely solely on the inner healer; she sought help from modern medicine as well as from complementary medicine and even explored spiritual paths and exercises.

Dagfrid has actively explored the process of her illness in terms of its social, psychic, and physical ramifications. The stories her illness needed to tell her resulted in healing and joy. She made her discoveries. She found her way.

A scientist in the sense of knowing and living her skill by experience, Dagfrid shares openly and candidly her life and discoveries with us. She has important things to say, and her book and her being in the world are invitations to join in and explore and enrich our own lives.

There is no doubt that illness is a stern teacher. But any illness has the power to show us its illusionary nature, and indeed it has the power to even teach us by experience the illusionary nature of death and separation itself.

Preface

Welcome, dear reader.

Life is one long process. There are always new things to learn. That is one of the exciting things about living.

Many years ago I was certain that I knew almost everything. Later on a lot of what I had thought of as truths were turned upside down.

Because what is truth?

I believed academic medicine and all scientific research were safely grounded in great wisdom and truth. Then, when I was confronted with a cancer diagnosis, my inner voice started to tell me otherwise.

The recent unveiling of false cancer research did not surprise me. Maybe it is just the tip of the iceberg as has been said several times in the media. This has also given me additional energy to come forward with my story based on what I have actually experienced in my own body.

I share everything I have learned about cancer because I have already experienced that some of my fellow humans could benefit from my experiences.

I have not been sitting here healthy today without the help of many people who have been with me during my journey. They have shared their wisdom and love and have supported me in my choices.

This led me to finding new strength within myself.

New insights came to me, and I have been able to leave behind the old ones that no longer are useful. My experiences have enabled me to grow, let me become truer and wiser. I have even become more closely connected with my own power.

In great love and humbleness I thank all the helpers and teachers who made my life possible and thereby helped to give me the pleasure of writing my story.

Thank you to my two sons who showed me their great love when I needed it most. Thank you to friends, family members, doctors, and the psychologist who, each in his or her own way, have contributed to help me to go on. They showed me new truths and supported me in my own choices on this magical journey that life is. One big thank you to the doctor I met in the middle of my cancer journey. She did not believe in my choice and thereby forced me to stand up for myself and to take responsibility for my own life.

This incident turned out to be very important for my entire cancer story—and for me.

My story was very complex. I had several shocks, one on top of the other. I had to process massive heaps of conflicts.

The best thing for me now is to live one day at the time, and today I am glad that I did not know how long it would take to work through all the shocks and conflicts.

It is also important for me to leave behind me the processes that I have been through. I must live as much as possible in present time. It has taken me a while to reconstruct my cancer story.

Modern cancer treatment is based on "fighting" and "killing." Most people feel fear just hearing the word *cancer*.

I believe in cooperation, even between our wonderful, wise, and beautiful bodies and souls, including cell abnormalities, life, and emotions. I do not believe in waging war. War only creates more war and is not life-supporting for us.

Taking a closer look at our fears can be valuable. We are often led by our fears without thinking through the situation closely. By getting in touch with our fears, breathing into them and feeling them, we can often cause the fear to just disappear ... like the many-headed troll. Then we have freedom to choose what we really like, and we are not controlled by fear. It is wonderful that, as humans, we can make choices. We need to remind ourselves about that and then use our courage to choose what feels right for us.

Aborigines of many cultures have always had simple ways of looking into the deep wisdom of the body, and these beliefs can lead to self-healing.

Good luck with your reading. Maybe you will discover many things that will turn your truths upside down. If so, it may be a good idea to put the book away, take a few deep breaths, and listen to what your own feelings are telling you. The answers to all the magical riddles of life are within you.

I invite you to make your own footprints.

Those who don't believe in magic will never find it.
—*Roald Dahl*

Part I

Dagfrid's cancer story

Dagfrid Kolaas

My first meeting with the cancer riddle

Life is a strange journey ...

Life takes us all to different directions ...

No one in my large family had ever experienced a cancer diagnosis; no one else that I knew had either. I thought about the issue of cancer as something scary and deadly and was well pleased to keep it at arm's length away from me. So much else was on my mind.

My interest in alternative thinking and understanding had been awakened already in the 1980s. I have always been interested in nature and have questioned the establishment. And I rarely put a pill in my mouth when something ailed me. I felt that something was wrong about doing that.

Love of life and all natural diversities grew through the 1990s. My interest in ecology, natural healing, and the meaning of life became stronger.

Many, many years ago I read the book *You Can Heal Your Life* by Louise L. Hay. The contents of the book fascinated me on all levels, and I was impressed by the whole life story of this woman. The most fascinating was her cancer story. She wrote about how she postponed her cancer operation and started to heal herself in different ways. The cancer disappeared, and there was nothing left to operate on. It seemed so obvious when I read it that I thought, *If ever I get cancer, I will do the same thing.*

Although the topic of cancer did not interest me at that point.

My personal meeting with the cancer issue

My interest in this issue was not awakened until one day in late summer of the year 2000. I had a tremendous relationship crisis. My marriage to my husband, after thirty-one years, was breaking down. It was a painful process.

We were living in the countryside on the west coast of Norway where we had founded a small eco-community together. It was close to paradise on earth, with our two sons; our friends; and happy, free-range animals. Most of my involvement was concentrated around the kids, the community, and the animals.

When the extent of the breakup dawned on me, I was shocked, and I broke down completely. I was unable to sleep, my hands and feet were constantly cold, and the pounds just dropped off. My thoughts were churning night and day without end. A small part of me was optimistic, but my soul was fatally wounded.

You gain strength, courage and confidence by every experience in which you really stop to look fear in the face. You are able to say to yourself, "I lived through this horror. I can take the next thing that comes along." You must do the thing you think you cannot do.
—Eleanor Roosevelt

On my own

I bought a small farm farther up on the west coast. I made big plans about building a small center there. I was born an optimist, so a part of me believed that all of the changes in my life would turn out well. At the same time, I knew I needed some time to process what had happened to me. Suddenly to be on my own after thirty-one years of marriage was difficult for me to deal with. Not seeing my teenager kids every day did not make it any better. I missed the animals and all of my close friends who still lived on the farm. Luckily I had my dog, Foxy, with me.

One day I felt two lumps in my right breast. I had felt lumps in my breasts earlier, several times during my periods and in connection with births and abortions. Therefore, those lumps didn't create any frustrations in me.

I came to mention it to a friend one day, and she talked me into having the lumps examined by my doctor.

When I visited my general practitioner, he referred me to the hospital for further examinations.

In a way, I was full to the rim, so this examination was no big deal for me. It was something that just piled on top of all the other things that were very tough and had given me such a hard time. It was not easy to really get in touch with all the emotions I was experiencing.

All lives holds difficulties that we are not prepared for.
Read and learn and prepare for life and healing.
—Bernard S. Siegel, MD

Tests at Haukeland Hospital

I asked a friend to come with me to the hospital on the day I would receive tests. I was not so cocky about the issue after all. The tests took time. I chose not to take mammography. I had done mammography once, and that was enough for me.

For some reason they asked me to come back several times for further testing. I began to understand that there could really be something wrong.

That sick feeling that clings to the walls in places like that began to crawl under my skin. It was a great relief when they finally were satisfied.

I believe in therapy instead of chemistry.
—*Dagfrid Kolaas*

Waiting period

It was a long time before the results of the tests came, but the waiting didn't worry me much. I had enough to do just keeping my head above water, because incredibly strong and painful feelings kept flooding in. I know now that I had experienced a severe shock when I first began to understand the consequences and the extent of the divorce. It was a huge task to cope with the feelings I was experiencing.

To shorten the wait, my friend and I went to visit good friends north of Bergen.

I received the cancer diagnosis through a call on my cell phone on the way to our destination. The strange thing was that I had suspected it, so it was no big surprise.

Fortunately it turned out to be okay visiting my friends with a brand new cancer diagnosis. They met me and respected me just the way I was feeling, and I did not have to put up a false face. Many deep, vulnerable, and honest talks followed over the next days and nights.

We don't see things as they are, we see them as we are.
—Anaïs Nin

Temptation to give up after a long life

I came to a point where I decided to give up, and it really suited me well. I was forty-six years old and had lived my life fully from day one. I felt I had experienced a lot … I had learned a lot.

So, when the diagnosis came I seriously contemplated simply giving up. I did not know if I had the guts to start carrying out my new dreams on my own. I almost saw the cancer diagnosis as a relief.

Another difficulty showed up at the same time. My job at the Bergen Incest Centre was terminated. It had been a temporary assignment, and all of my other work had been on our farm.

For several years I had studied and delved into the topic of death. I had taken mental journeys into previous lifetimes and also into "life" between lives. I had been a regression therapist and had followed many of my clients on their journeys into former lives.

I had no fear of death; rather, I played with the thought and found it really tempting. Just then I was more afraid of life, and afraid that the spark of life should never return to me. It was totally gone.

I began to plan where I wanted to go and live for the time I had left to live. I did not want to bother anyone with my illness. I wanted to make the transition as painless as possible.

When you think everything is someone else's fault, you
will suffer a lot. When you realize that everything springs
only from yourself, you will learn both peace and joy.
—*Dalai Lama*

Love and miracles

Something happened. My younger son at age thirteen understood that it was really possible to die of cancer, and also that I was about to give up. Weeping, he threw his arms around me, sobbing. Again and again he said, "Mom, you're not allowed to die!"

This was a strong experience for me. My inner life had been in total darkness and death ever since the crisis engulfed me, but now a tiny ember of life began to glow again.

Some days later my older son repeated the message: "Mom, don't give up! I need you. I love you. And I miss you so much at home!" Then I decided to choose life. The situation was turned upside down again.

Yes, Dagfrid, what do you do now? I felt incredibly worn out. I had no strength to carry out my old pattern: be a good girl, pull up your sleeves, and get on with it!

For a long time I have had a good rapport with my inner voice, and I knew I had invisible helpers following me. I opened up to great trust and gained peace in my soul.

I began to pray for help. I asked to be led to exactly what I needed.

We must remove the word impossible *from our vocabulary.*
Whoever does not believe in miracles is not a realist.
—*Bernie S. Siegel.*

What makes me want to live?

The most important thing for me now was to regain my spark of life and to work through those painful feelings that had almost paralyzed me day and night.

It was difficult for me to sleep. I had no appetite and felt cold all the time. It seemed there was nowhere for me to hide and get some peace. It felt as if all the walls had fallen, and I was left there naked feeling totally petrified. My low self-esteem only increased, and my longing for my old life and the kids almost drove me crazy.

I had previously gotten to know the psychologist Rune Amundsen and his wife Grethe, who lived in Sogn. I had come to know them both as broad-minded and nonjudgmental and truly loving.

I made an appointment for therapy with Rune.

We begin immediately on the phone, as he lived quite some distance away. It was difficult to begin processing the most vulnerable feelings alone, so getting this help was priceless.

Many strange synchronicities began to happen.

I recalled the story told by Louise L. Hay. After they found a tumor, she postponed the recommended surgery for three months. During that time Louise did several things. The most important, as I see it, was that she processed the hurting emotions and decided to love herself more. I had never heard about anyone else who had taken a natural path to heal cancer.

The very same week that I was given my diagnosis, another ground-breaking book was released. I received four independent calls from friends: "Dagfrid, you just *have* to read this book!" I understood it had to be important, so I went right out and bought *The Journey: A Practical Guide to Healing Your Life and Setting Yourself Free* by Brandon Bays.

Brandon Bays had a cancerous tumor in her abdomen that was the size of a football. She did the same thing that Louise L. Hay did—she postponed surgery, started to treat her emotions (among other things), and the cancer disappeared. There was nothing left to operate on.

This was incredibly inspiring.

When one door of happiness closes, another opens; but often we look so long at the closed door that we do not see the one which has been opened for us.
—Helen Keller

Excellent helpers at the hospital

I was assigned to a very broad-minded and loving surgeon at the hospital. I was still so shattered that I dared not go for only a fully natural treatment, so we agreed to go for an in-between solution. The lumps would be removed at the hospital. If something more should occur with the cancer, then I would handle it with natural treatment.

In a way I was relieved. I knew only about those two writers from the United States—Louise Hay and Brandon Bays—who had done it! They were a bit far away ...

I calmed down with our agreement.

Then I meet a friend who reminded me that I could choose breast-preserving surgery if I wanted to! She told me that many women had woken up in shock, finding themselves with one breast missing. No one had told them beforehand that the breast could be saved.

Oh my God! This was news for me. I had been certain that all they were planning to do was removing the two lumps in my breast.

Yes, my helpers certainly appeared at the right time.

There is only one journey. Going inside yourself.
—Rainer Maria Rilke

Angels, do they exist?

A great angel showed up on my path. She understood how terribly hard it was for me to live alone for the first time in my life. Well, my dog, Foxy, was with me, my very special dog who was a great helper in his own special way. But I really missed somebody to live with.

My friend took care of that. She offered to come and stay with me until the world felt like a better place to be in and live in.

Thanks, and again thanks!

When the day of the operation arrived I actually felt peace. I felt confident that I would get the help I needed, and that it would be a good experience.

I had my favorite music playing during the operation.

The doctor also respected my special diet. I brought two full bags of health food supplies. Everybody working at the hospital appeared to be just angels. I think the work I did on my fear about the hospital had some influence on this experience.

All the time, I was aware that self-love was something I needed to give time and attention to. I was advised not to socialize with other cancer patients, because they tend to delve into fear and horror stories about cancer. That might not be so good for me in my vulnerable state.

At the hospital, I stayed in bed much of the time, listened to music, and "felt myself to the rim" with all the people sending me flowers and coming to visit me and calling me. I closed my eyes and visualized my heart filled up with all this. It worked wonders for me. I felt able to receive the love! Wonderful. The inner peace and love increased. The darkness and painful feelings in my inner world began to dissolve.

Yes, I was actually making choices about what I allowed to influence me.

For years I had realized that the way the various media communicate news and other information often depressed me. I was used to choosing to stay away from things that weren't good for me. Now that I was feeling so fragile, it was even more important to protect myself.

Something unexpected happens

The doctor told me that the surgery had gone well. They had also re-moved fourteen lymphatic nodes just in case! I became very puzzled. Why had I not been informed of this and asked about it beforehand? The final result of the operation would be revealed at my next checkup. I felt incredibly tired. So much drama in such a short time. The doctor recommended convalescence.

I chose the Tonsaasen Sanatorium as the best place. They served good vegetarian food there, which was my main diet at the time. And I had a good feeling about the place.

There was not an opening at Tonsaasen for some weeks, so after I left the hospital, I continued my deep and honest process.

I also experienced a troublesome physical reaction. The spot where the lumps had been in my breast filled up with liquid. Not just a little, but a lot. The breast was engorged and hurting terribly. No one had explained to me that this is common. I was told about it when I called the hospital a few days later. I went several times back to the hospital to have the liquids drained out.

I carefully observed my dreams. I had often been able to gain under-standing about difficulties through dreams.

I continued the sessions with Rune. I felt very isolated, and Rune helped me to get more in touch with myself and also to open up and connect with the outer world. It felt good to get help with the things I felt I couldn't do by myself. Therapy helped me emotionally and in interpreting my dreams.

I also went to the hairdresser. Fixing up the exterior when the inside doesn't feel too good can also be a therapy. At the salon I found a folder from the Maharishi Ayurveda Health Center outside of Lillehammer. I immediately felt this place was a good fit for me, so I cancelled Tonsaasen.

Turn your wounds into wisdom.

—*Oprah Winfrey*

Treatment for body and soul

Soon I found myself on the train to Lillehammer. At the clinic I received wonderful massages every day, something that felt vitally important to me in these lonely times without much contact with others.

I participated in meditation groups and ate organic food. There was colon cleansing every day.

The landscape of the village of Mesnalia was beautiful and the perfect place for taking walks.

One of the doctors at the centre was schooled in both ayurvedic medicine and traditional medicine. He shared my view on cancer. The ayurvedic treatment of cancer includes treatment of the emotions. It also includes diet, herbs, and other things.

This turned out to be ten fine and recreational days for me, although I missed the kids terribly while I was there. On the other hand it felt good not to have to keep track of them, because I was often depressed. I cried a lot during these days. I also missed my former life on the farm.

You move totally away from reality when you believe
that there is a legitimate reason to suffer.
—*Byron Katie*

An interesting coincidence

Back home in Bergen again, the time came for my first checkup after surgery. I had recovered so much that I felt I could go to the appointment alone.

I was to see a doctor I hadn't seen before. She was young and very proud of her academic medicine. She told me that they had found an area of about 8.5 centimeters of abnormal cell structures in my right breast (ductal carcinoma in situ). They had already arranged to operate and remove my breast in a few days.

I told her that I had decided to move on with natural treatment, an agreement I had made with my former surgeon—and with myself.

Now I felt strong enough to stand by such a decision. She didn't like what I was saying. "Then you must accept chemotherapy, radiation, and hormonal treatment," she told me.

In the meantime I had read about the side effects of those treatments so I politely turned down this offer as well.

The doctor obviously found me to be an impudent patient and began to get agitated. I began to cry. Things were getting really wild. She ran out of her office, and after a while she returned with a piece of paper with words typed on it. I was still in tears.

A life-changing experience

The young doctor handed me the document she had written and asked me to sign it. It verified that I had rejected all further treatment and that I had to take 100 percent responsibility for my own life.

She said, hysterically, "Now the alternative therapists are going to cheat you and take all your money. You will get a full spreading, and you are going straight to your death!"

At this, I felt she had gone too far. I told her that her reaction was abusive.

She laid the document in front of me.

Something strange happened in that very moment.

I stopped crying …

A power was welling up inside me. It filled me up as I signed … I was taking responsibility for my own life!

From that moment on I knew everything was going to be all right.

Yes, quite simply, I was feeling happy.

I had experienced a very short interval between feeling catastrophic and feeling powerful.

> *Be the change that you wish to see in the world.*
> —*Mahatma Gandhi*

Now what?

"Yes, and now what, Dagfrid?" Safely outside the gates of the hospital I sat down on a bench and lit up a long-missed cigarette.

I still wanted not to struggle. I didn't want to go back to that old "good girl" pattern of mine. I was just too tired. I also knew there must be other ways to meet the challenges.

I went back to praying—for help from the invisible and visible helpers.

I made up my mind that if I was still meant to be here on earth, I would get all the help I needed.

I prayed that only those who would support my choice of natural treatment would get in touch with me. Support was what was most important for me now.

In a way I was putting my life into the hands of the Universe, and I promised to do my part. I envisioned that "my part" was going to be done with ease, love, and so much joy that I would be able to manage.

I know God will not give me anything I can't handle.
I just wish that He didn't trust me so much.
—Mother Teresa

My prayers are heard

Many people knew that I was going to have this post-op checkup. They waited with anticipation for the results. I had a strong feeling that many would be scared by what I had to tell them.

Previously I had been able to feel in my body when somebody was feeling sorry for me. I have felt how the energy disappeared and left me powerless. Now it was important that nobody should be worried about my choice.

Miracles happen. Only the ones who turned out to support me came through on my phone once I turned it on again.

I planned a treatment with color-light therapy. The next gift waited for me there. A good friend greeted me and told me that he'd had leukemia as a young man. He had chosen to go deeply into his emotions rather than going to academic medicine for help.

Not long afterwards he had been completely healed. This had been many years ago. So this angel showed up with this wonderful sentence to me: "Congratulations, you have just given yourself a great gift today."

It warmed me to the core of my soul.

In addition to that, the light treatment on my breast was very soothing. This man was completely void of fear of cancer and full of pride on my behalf.

God and breasts

I had previously accepted an invitation to dinner at a friend's house that same evening. Of course I shared with her the powerful experiences of that day. She was also without fear about the situation and exclaimed, "You know, Dagfrid, if it had been me, I would have told God, 'If you really mean that I am supposed to wander on this earth with only one breast, you'd better take me back home again!'"

We had a lot of good laughs. And this itself was powerful medicine.

I was calm and confident in my choice. I maintained a strong feeling that I had made the right decision.

I supported this decision by reminding myself about the first surgeon I had consulted. She had given me her full support in choosing my own alternative ways—if the cancer should still be there.

> *Life is a gift. Every challenge is a gift in the end. Getting cancer was a gift for me. If your challenge doesn't feel like a gift, you haven't reached to the end yet.*
> —*Anita Moorjani*

What can I do myself?

Yes, Dagfrid, I told myself, *it is now it really matters and your main task is to get well.* It was what I had promised my kids.

I was on sick leave at the time. The kids lived mostly with their father, and so I had plenty of time to go into the study of cancer healing.

I monitored my dreams, listening for possible messages they might communicate to me—and often they did. Also I paid attention to occurrences of unplanned events I encountered along my way. I was busy with these and other occupations, but I was still a bit insecure about what else to do.

Intuition was my greatest helper. I spent a lot of time in silence, breathing deeply and listening. I was confident that I was being led in the right direction. You know the expression, all roads lead to Rome. This was my truth. I was sure I would find my way.

I felt that breathing was my most important tool. To breathe all the way down, into the pit of my stomach and thereby provide the cells and my blood with new and fresh energy. This was life rejuvenating.

My body needed this when it was going to kick off its completely unique program of self-healing.

Joy and deep breaths are maybe the most important tools when the body is "on the job" of getting well again.

I felt I needed to set boundaries against anything that did not lift me up. I further restricted information from the media, especially all news on television, in newspapers, and on radio. For a while I watched only uplifting and humorous programs. I watched the television series *Around Norway*, a wonderful show that focuses mainly on positive and simple things in ordinary people's lives around the country.

Too bad good news doesn't sell. At least not yet.

Nature was very important to me. Being outside in God's free nature was really balm to my soul. Sitting on a stump in the woods, hugging a tree, walking in the mountains and the forests and fields—all of it was pure medicine. I enjoyed birdsong and the cycles of nature. I took advantage of this as often as I could.

Being near water is very cleansing. Sitting by the seaside, by a mountain lake, or by a river, one can let all painful emotions emerge and be expressed. Then they can be released into the water. These were things that worked well for me.

I sat in my favorite chair and listened to soothing and beautiful music, preferably at full blast so I could feel it penetrating my body down to the cellular level.

Fire is also transformational. A fireplace vendor said to me, "Fireplaces should be given to people and be covered by the health services." I totally agreed. Sitting in front of the fire when I need supplies of soothing and good energy feels good.

There is something magical about the forces of nature. Looking into an open flame and feeling the warmth from the fire goes under my skin.

In my experience it is important not to push away or deny the troublesome and painful emotions. You have to confront them. Thinking only positive thoughts may be negative, because the painful emotions need to be "met" before they can be released. To suppress them is not a good solution.

After you release the painful emotions, it is important to be aware of what you focus on.

I spend a lot of time focusing on the healthy parts of my life. I didn't think about the cancer; rather, I thought about all the things about me that were healthy and everything that was positive in my life All the time my main focus was that I would get well.

This has become an important topic further on in my life too. It is easy to be drawn into drama through television and other media.

I think it's important to know about the problems in the world. It is useful information. That being said, I think it's more important not to focus too much on all those dramatic issues; otherwise, it is easy to experience life with fear.

I chose not to have television, newspapers, and magazines. Now I choose, by using the Internet and books, what I want to focus on. I am grateful to everyone who is sharing topics through these media that provide inspiration and hope. *Thanks.*

> *I will not be distracted by noise, chatter, or setbacks.*
> *Patience, commitment, grace, and purpose will guide me.*
> —*Louise L. Hay*

The Health House in Sogn

I felt that I would not go to any of the famous natural healing centers for cancer like Santa Monica in Poland, Vidarklinikken in Sweden, or Humlegaarden in Denmark.

The main thing for me was to work with the emotional issues, then diet. Other things came second.

For me, it was appropriate going to Villa Magnolia, a Health House that psychologist Rune Amundsen and his wife Grethe had opened in a wonderful villa on the west coast of Norway. I took my dog, Foxy, with me and drove up there. It turned out to be just what I needed at the time:

This place provided alleviation and processing for all of Dagfrid.

I received massages from Grethe. Often I felt "dead" in this lonely time, and being touched was miraculous.

The community and wonderful meetings with other people who had signed in there worked wonders.

The good talks with Rune allowed me to enter deeply into my feelings and were gold to me. My journeys into the deep on Rune's bench really helped me in the process with the painful emotions. Still, feelings of hatred, rage, jealousy, envy, poor-me, and so on emerged. Getting help to go deeply was a great gift.

Vividly I recall one day when I met a Light on my inner journey. The Light presented himself as Jesus. He filled me with light, and I was given an incredible inner peace. Then all the other people involved in my crisis emerged, and I was given an explanation from the Light as to why this had to happen in my life: When the transformation of these painful feelings was through, I would see the transformation as a great gift to me.

I was filled with feelings of forgiveness and joy. The Light (Jesus) further explained, that I had chosen this situation to grow, and as a result I would obtain access to even more light, compassion, and love …

Actually it was not so easy meeting this Light, because as a young woman I had turned my back on the church. But now, the time was obviously right for a new meeting.

This experience is uplifting and meaningful to me even to this day.

I am a realist. I expect miracles.
—*Dr. Wayne W. Dyer*

Experience results in expertise

Living and cooking together with other people at the Health House was a great gift. The fellowship emerging in this kind of situation was therapy in itself. Several were in deep crises, but a fellowship like this was easing the burden. Most of the people who sought this kind of help wished to release the pain without medication.

"Illness is the body's attempt to heal you". is one of Rune's words of wisdom.

And another one is: "Listen to your inner doctor. Deep inside yourself you will find the answers for healing."

One of the first things he said to me after I got the cancer diagnosis was: "Exciting—now you will become a cancer expert, because everyone who has been through an illness learns what it really is. And then, Dagfrid, you can help others who are confronted with this diagnosis, because you will have experienced it in your own body, not just read about it or met somebody else who has had cancer."

The nice thing about both Rune and Grethe is that they never "see" the illness that people have. They look straight through it and straight at the growth that comes when a person has lived through a situation.

Rune's singing and his joy in playing the guitar made certain that there always was such *joy of life* "clinging to the walls" at Villa Magnolia. Grethe's big heart, delightful humor, and great singing voice added even more to this.

I spent two weeks there, and it was worth gold.

It was a treasure for me and all others "inmates" that I had been able to bring my dog Foxy with me. Foxy could always "feel" when somebody was in extra pain, and he often would follow a person in pain and lie down really close to him or her, even at night.

There was no one there in white uniforms. We were the experts, each one an expert on his or her own crisis, and we helped each other enormously. We knew where the shoe was tight. It really didn't take much to release the pain.

The body has an amazing ability to be well in itself. We have a built-in self-diagnostic system that surpasses all electronics that have so far been produced. Once we have set our own diagnose we start to correct the imbalances. Sometimes we need a little assistance in this work.
—*Dr. Magnar Kleiven*

Oh, that Jesus!

During my childhood I had a kind of traumatic relationship with the church and consequently Jesus too. He disappeared from my life.

The incident with the Light gave me a new opinion about Jesus.

I got a picture of him, one that was said to have its origin in the Shroud of Turin. It radiated a strong and confident energy, and that picture became of great importance to me from then on.

I kept it on my nightstand during the night and in the middle of the kitchen table during the day.

It looked like power and healing was coming out through the eyes of Jesus. I was helped by this divine radiance, especially when I missed the kids so much that I was almost turning mad.

It is unbelievable that it worked, but it did!

My favorite quote:

> *Let the one among you who is without sin be the first to cast a stone.*
> —*Jesus Christ*

Friends are like diamonds

I can't say that enough. Friends meant everything during these tough times. Some of the old ones disappeared along the way of the crisis.

Divorce and cancer together made a heavy combination, and it was not always easy for friends to relate to what I was going through. And I understood that. I have experienced situations myself in which I felt it difficult to meet somebody who was in deep crisis.

Luckily, I had friends who were not afraid, and more new friends appeared. To be seen and listened to during this time was of tremendous value. I felt that the love of friends was contributing to my healing.

Sometimes I need to vent my problems with somebody in order to be able to solve my conflicts. Maybe there is greater value in this than we realize.

We have made a kind of an "expert" society in which we are convinced that we must go to, for instance, a psychologist to talk about a crisis. But the value of being listened to and fully accepted by good friends may be just as valuable.

Nothing in life is to be feared, it is only to be understood.
Now is the time to understand more, so that we may fear less.
—*Marie Curie*

Next checkup

I called the hospital to say that I didn't want to meet with the young doctor who had tried to scare me into removing my breast. I asked to see the first surgeon I had met. I would wait until she returned. The receptionist understood and set up a new consultation with my first surgeon.

At the consultation, she examined the breast on the surface, and there was no sign of new cancerous lumps. I'd had a feeling about that for a while already, because the joy of life was coming back more and more, and days went on without the past overtaking me.

I had actually felt healthy for a long time. I enjoyed good food and drink and had put on some weight. I was sleeping better than I had been able to for a long time, and my body felt nicely warm again. I felt that an inner peace was growing.

> *Don't let the behavior of others destroy your inner peace.*
> —*Dalai Lama*

All those miraculous cures

For years I had used my food as my medicine. I ate organic food, and my meat came from free-range, happy animals.

All my life I have had trouble swallowing pills. Deep inside I did not actually believe in them.

After I got the cancer diagnosis, I let myself be convinced by well-meaning authors and high-sounding therapists, and I began to use a lot of supplements.

After a while I felt that I was putting stuff in my mouth because somebody else had told me it was healthy. Maybe it was not a good idea after all. I even found totally contradicting advice for the same type of cancer.

It was not easy to make sense of all this.

I decided to throw away all the vitamin supplements, the minerals, the shark cartilage—all of it.

From then on it was my inner voice guiding me, and it was pleasure. My gut feeling took the lead: "Eat and drink what you prefer, Dagfrid. The body tells you what you need."

A totally new freedom was mine.

Gosh, it felt sooo good …

Common sense is very uncommon.
—*Horace Greeley*

My life as a city person

A year after the initial crisis, I moved to Bergen. I wanted to be more available to my boys. Besides, after a long life as a country girl, I felt excited to check out what the city had to offer.

Before the move, I had changed doctors and had begun seeing a holistic doctor in Bergen. It was a really good thing to do. He was extremely supportive and told me to choose my own way.

In addition to my own choices of natural therapies, he suggested that I take mistletoe. I managed to smuggle it in from Stockholm through a good friend. Then I learned to give myself injections, something I never had thought possible. But halfway into the cure, when the amount was increased, I felt very sick, and we decided to break off the mistletoe cure.

Then I felt really healthy again and wanted to get back to work. My doctor asked me to wait for a while. "You have never been out of work because of illness before, and this is a brilliant opportunity to really get to know yourself and to learn the value of just 'being.' All your life you have been there for others."

I had never had so much time for only myself. It was a new situation, and I was not familiar with it. It was scary at times, but slowly and steadily I found the deeper value in it.

The most important thing was self-love—loving myself and being able to receive help and love from others. Being valuable as a human person without doing or working much was a new truth that came to me slowly.

It was difficult for "doing-Dagfrid" to decide what I really wanted to do just for myself.

I often felt selfish, but others told me that in a situation like this it was common. The comfort I was given was: self-love has nothing to do with egoism.

Very interesting, but challenging, too, at the same time.

I am willing to release the need to be unworthy. I am worthy of the
very best in life, and I now lovingly allow myself to accept it.
—*Louise L. Hay*

Art therapy

When the crisis struck I was in the middle of training to become an art therapist. This was a Danish education course that extended over two and a half years. It had been established in Norway in 1999.

The course included introductions into many of the different ways of alternative thinking, like shamanism, psycho-drama, breath therapy, dream interpretation, liberation through painting, spirituality and dance, group processes, depth psychology, and much, much more.

The curriculum was based on Jung's psychology, and there were a lot of books to be read. What a gift I was given at this school. At the same time, I really got to learn a lot of practical psychology—by going through a crisis myself.

During our training we learned to feel in the body what was going on rather than "learning" through only the intellect. It was obvious that we would be better therapists when we had cleared our own problems and emotions.

We had thirteen weeks all together of tutoring, and during that time all of us stayed together. I made good friends among those seventeen women from all parts of Norway. Sharing with them was a great bonus.

*Don't walk behind me; I may not lead. Don't walk in front of
me; I may not follow. Just walk beside me and be my friend.*
—Albert Camus

Pen pal

In the school of art therapy I met a wonderful woman from the island of Hitra on the west coast. She loved to write. We developed strong ties, and soon letters appeared in my mailbox. I was reluctant to answer, because this new friend of mine was a school principal. I knew my writing contained many errors. Did I dare to write her back?

After a long period of inner persuasion and deep breathing, I dove into it. It turned out to be the beginning of a long and wonderful pen pal friendship. I was happy to find that even this angel made typos. Then I relaxed and could write straight from the heart whatever passed through my fingers.

We started sharing our nightly dreams and our thoughts about life as it goes on. I felt infinitely good to receive responses from her, as my self-esteem was hanging on one brittle tread at that time.

Soon it became evident to me that writing about my difficulties was powerful therapy. I actually felt better the minute I posted a letter. Yes, a negative feeling that is shared loses some of its power. And, of course, her letters often arrived at those moment when I was really feeling low and needed that sort of "vitamin shot."

The teacher who is indeed wise does not bid you to enter the house of his wisdom but rather leads you to the threshold of your mind.
—Khalil Gibran

Relapse

About one year after my crises started, I woke up one day finding myself in deep crisis again—it was as if the breakup of my marriage had just happened. I did everything I could to take myself out of the feeling: I breathed, meditated, painted, and went for walks, but nothing helped.

The worst thing about it was the feeling of being defeated. Had none of the processing of the painful emotions worked at all? All the discussions, all the therapy, all the healing sessions and …

The feelings were stuck like a knot in my gut, and the physical pain just kept getting worse and worse.

I got hold of painkillers and took them, but just vomited them out again. In the end I went to the emergency ward, and they sent me to hospital.

I was well received, and a strange thing happened when I was being put to bed and tucked in nicely—the pain dissolved!

I got to talk to a young, sympathetic doctor and we decided that it had all been "just the nerves."

The next day, when I returned home, a letter was waiting for me in the mailbox. A good friend had been to an alternative healing fair in Oslo where she had met a man from Switzerland. He had lectured about the natural curing of cancer, and he had brought along an interview with Dr. Ryke Geerd Hamer.

And now I had it in my hand!

You can read the interview with Dr. Hamer on this website: http://www.newmedicine.ca/interview.php

My best moment in bed

I went straight to bed. Even though I was still worn out from two days and nights of horrible pain, I started to read.

In the interview Dr. Hamer described the natural reactions in the body when cancer appears and what bodily reactions follow naturally—both in the crisis phase, and in the healing phase.

This was powerful stuff. I was reading about myself!

I recognized the signs I had experienced in my body when the cancer was discovered: no appetite, trouble sleeping, buzzing thoughts, cold hands and feet. He also concluded that cancer came on the aftermath of a tough and often shocking experience.

I read and read till my eyes were literally wide and wet. Then I reached the chapter about symptoms in the healing phase. Here I recognized my own experiences—as things begin to get back to normal, there will be a feeling of deep inner peace, the body will be warmer, and sleep and appetite will improve.

Then this German doctor explained that some complications might occur in the middle of the healing phase. One possibility was that the patient could suddenly feel as if the crisis had just happened, and the emotions could be just as strong as when the crisis actually did happen.

Gosh! That was exactly what just had happened to me! Then I really cried, but it was tears of joy.

I read the interview through, several times.

This has been the most important information in my life so far.

The New Medicine

A German medical doctor, Dr. Ryke Geerd Hamer, who was born in 1934, experienced the death of his son. His son was in a shooting accident and died later in his father's arms. Later both the doctor and his wife, also a doctor, were diagnosed with cancer. This sparked the doctor's thoughts about the cancers. Was it incidental that the cancer emerged just then?

Could the onset of the cancers be connected to his son's death in some way?

Three years later he was employed as the leader of the internal medicine section at a gynecological cancer ward at the University of Munich. He had the opportunity to look for similarities in other cases and compare them with his own experience. Had these patients been exposed to conflicts and shocks, and could their cancer have been caused by this? He was really surprised to find that his theory proved to be correct.

All of the patients had had at least one strong emotional experience just before the appearance of their cancer, and most of their physical reactions were similar; for instance, the loss of sleep at night, cold hands and feet, weight loss, and so on. The doctor was happy that he had discovered this, because it was completely new to conventional medical opinion.

When he shared this discovery with his colleagues he was asked to either forget everything he had discovered so far or resign from the university clinic.

The universe is full of magical things patiently waiting upon us to be wiser.
—Eden Phillpots

I need to learn more!

I got high reading this information. I felt that I just had to learn more about the discoveries this man had made.

I got in touch with the people who had translated the interview with Dr. Hamer into Norwegian, and wonder of wonders—in just a short time there would be a course about this issue in Oslo.

I rearranged my calendar, packed my suitcase … and I was super happy.

Harald Baumann, Dr. Hamer's right hand through many years, had arrived from Switzerland. And we were an assembly of curious people from all over the country. I sat down on the first row with open mind and senses.

It turned out to be a lot of news about the cancer issue. Dr. Hamer had continued the research on his own, and he was still finding new insights. For instance, he discovered that all the people who had cancer in the same organ had had similar traumatic experiences before the cancer appeared

Awesome! This was really news for me. Baumann mentioned, as an example, that if a right-handed women experiences something traumatic and shocking, something totally surprising with the part-ner—often a divorce—then the cancer often appears in the right breast!

I was right-handed, I had gone through a traumatic divorce, and I'd had cancer in my right breast!

So many completely new insights turned up during the weekend that I felt as though my head would crack. But I was jubilant. I felt as if I had always known this.

Why had nobody taken interest in the research of this doctor? Even those alternative institutes in our neighboring countries had closed their eyes to the emotional and conflict part of the cancer issue.

I could feel my energy rising.

This knowledge had to be shared with everyone who would listen and who wanted to learn about new cancer research!

One should not ignore the fact that in a few decades very much of today's technology and chemical treatment of disease will be scrapped because we get an acknowledgment, even amongst the so-called experts, that man has many more abilities than anyone previously thought.
—Dr. Magnar Kleiven

CT scan

In the interview with Dr. Hamer I read how he could interpret a person's bodily status, or what she or he had been through, by studying pictures of the brain.

He discovered that when a dramatic situation occurs, three things happens at the same time:

1. The situation creates a certain strong emotion.

2. The emotion is reflected in the corresponding area of the brain.

3. Cellular changes occur in the organ that is controlled by this brain area.

So three areas are involved at the same time: the emotions, the brain, and an organ.

I'd had a computed tomography scan (CT scan) of my brain before I went to Oslo. During his time with Dr. Hamer, Harald Bauman had learned how to interpret CT brain images. And now he could interpret mine!

I was really excited. He put the CT image of my brain on an over-head projector and started to tell me about my life. Before he began, he knew nothing about me, but I found myself sitting there gaping. He told me about different significant experiences in my life since childhood.

He was able to tell me that I had had cancer in my right breast, but now it was healed! Everything he said was exactly right.

When we have powerful experiences our brain is affected. This means that all powerful emotional experiences leave marks on the brain. It sounds so logical. Why hasn't anybody thought about this before?

Arranging workshops

I asked Baumann if he was willing to come to Bergen to share Hamer's research. He loved to teach everyone who was ready for this new understanding, so his answer was a big yes.

Readily and with great joy, I started handing out the interview with Dr. Hamer, and began gathering people together for workshops.

I cooperated with others, and soon we had contact with a few people who were interested, and Harald Baumann came.

Again I was back in the classroom ready to learn even more. In Oslo there had been so much new knowledge at one time, it was impossible to absorb all of it.

It was exciting to share this with many of my good friends. Being the only person in Bergen who had heard about this breakthrough knowledge would have made me feel lonely.

Once you start believing that something is possible, you start to let
it into your awareness, and then it start to become true for you.
—Anita Moorjani

Could the spread of cancer be caused by new conflicts?

I was ready to absorb yet another brand-new truth. If a shock or conflict is what makes us get cancer, then what about proliferation?

I had wondered about why cancer, when it spread, didn't attack the organs and areas close by. That would seem natural according to my old beliefs.

Did a new cancer in another place develop because of a new shock? Hmmm, this was really something. It actually sounded sensible. My intuition told me the same too. But then what was going on?

I was very vulnerable when I got cancer. In this situation I was very susceptible to new shocks.

Most people have great fear of cancer, so getting a diagnosis could just possibly trigger a new conflict and a new shock.

The research shows that lung cancer often develops as a reaction to the fear of death. People who have lung cancer often have received an initial diagnosis of cancer in another area.

Why have so many nonsmokers developed lung cancer? I wondered. All the pieces seemed to fall into place.

Like a waving of the magic wand, all of my fear of cancer spreading disappeared from my life.

Little me ... or?

Dr. Hamer continued his research and he has come to the conclusion:

All cancer patients he had investigated had had a shock before their cancer showed up, and everyone with similar emotional experiences got cancer in the same area or organ in the body.

This really brings up a lot of thoughts about today's cancer treatments. I have not yet heard of doctors talking about the emotional aspect of the treatment. And what about modern cancer research at incalculable costs?

For many years, I had both experienced and seen the connection between emotions, thoughts, and illnesses. But now I really began to realize that this applies to cancer also.

What is keeping academic medicine from making this connection?

Could it be that little me actually understand something that the modern doctors of today still have not opened up to?

What I do know is that my choice of treatment saved the Norwegian state between one and two million Norwegian kroner, and I have mostly been bullied for doing it.

Why is it that none of the doctors has invited me in and asked me how I became healthy? One fine day I am sure such collaboration will come.

I feel very proud; I still have my right breast hanging there. I don't know how I would have coped with walking around with just one. I honor all who do.

Cancer cells

As long as I can remember, I had thought that all of us live with harmful cancer cells in our bodies. In special situations these dangerous cells could get out of control, and I have been amply warned over the years by "experts"—certain foods, certain lifestyles, cigarettes, and genes could be dangerous.

Now I understand more. We don't have any "ambushing cells." When we experience shock or sudden unexpected trauma, that emotional experience can trigger a cell change in the body.

Cells cannot get out of control. All cellular changes are programmed to help us find a solution to a crisis, and partly to repair the body when the crisis is over.

Dr. Hamer calls this the Devine Intelligence of the cells. In Spanish his research is called *La Medicina Segrada*—the Sacred Medicine.

When we have solved the conflict, then fungi, viruses, and bacteria move in and make the body healthy again.

So simple.

I am really looking forward to a time when academic medicine will start to take an interest in this.

My new mission

A new meaning entered into my life. The discovery of different ways to look at the cancer issue was big for me.

I wanted to share this with others who were not willing to settle down with the existing understanding of cancer. It felt super-important to me to make known the fact that we do have choices when a cancer diagnosis comes up.

Some people think that they must do as the doctors say. It is important for me to inform you that we have the legal right to choose what treatment we want to trust.

I continued to gather people for workshops with Harald Baumann. We held more classes, both in Oslo and in Bergen.

It was a great inspiration for me to do this. There was great interest among many people to gain insight into this pioneering research. It brought meaning and joy to my life, as the research agreed with my inner feeling of how the enigma of cancer had been put together.

Dr. Hamer had arrived at an even more exact overview of cancer. This overview was far more detailed than the index developed by Louise L. Hay.

Yes, this just had to be shared with others.

When Harald Baumann was in Bergen, he stayed at my house, and I got ample opportunity to ask more questions about this incredible research.

Advice to cancer patients

I am often asked what I recommend to people who are in the midst of their cancer experience. It is very important for me to weigh my words, because we are all unique. So I make several suggestions and ask them to listen to their own feelings for what is right for them.

If they feel fear about going the natural path, maybe it is right for them to take the path of academic medicine. It does not exclude taking an active part in the healing.

So why not: "Yes please, both, thank you!"

All of us have emotions, both negative and positive. It is totally all right that they are there. The important thing here is saying "yes" to open up to the emotions, feel what they are, and talk about them, especially the painful ones.

Help is often needed here, because one of the experiences of the cancer patient may be a feeling of emotional isolation and having a perception that this can't be shared with anybody.

The feeling that no one can understand just what they have experienced and felt in the stressful situation can be strong. Many have rage, hatred, feelings of "poor me," among others, and they find it impossible to process them. My experience is that it is absolutely possible to process all of them, but the person must, of course, be willing to actively approach them.

Another thing of great importance is that there is often more than one conflict to be solved. This is where good counseling becomes extremely valuable.

Everyone must take his or her own choices, but it is of great value to have somebody wise to talk with. Sometimes it may be enough to solve a conflict practically.

Physical pain is a sensitive issue. I have experienced many times myself that by breathing into the pain it has disappeared. Pain is often connected with fear.

It saddens me that morphine is used too often to ease the pain of cancer patients. My experience is that morphine paralyses feelings, and it is so important to grasp the emotions of fear and to delve into them deeply.

There are many possibilities for doing this. It can be done with a trusted friend, a family member, or in a therapy setting.

Self-love is important. Use this unique opportunity to really get to know yourself. Listen to what you really need, and maybe learn to say "no." Set some boundaries and learn to receive from others. The last point I feel applies to everyone I have talked to.

Regarding diets and food, I don't want to give advice. It is a confusing issue for most people in this phase. Magazines are full of advice and sensational cures. Concerning cancer there are even contradictory opinions. Our personal truth also influences the food that we eat. The most important thing is to make sure that pleasure and enjoyment accompany food and drink. This affects the whole body positively. If you believe strongly in a diet, yes, then it becomes right for you.

Stress and food do not go well together.

I have been through many truths about what kind of food is right. Now I eat and drink what feels good for me, and then mostly organic food.

Nowadays I am not working as a therapist any longer, but I love to share my story.

Hope and support

It is very important not to take hope away from people.

As long as there is life, there is hope.

I have met many who were given up on by academic medicine. It is easier to give help then, because both the cancer patient and the family are ready to make different choices.

One gift we can give ourselves is a great hope.

Creating hope gives us strength to start the self-healing processes in the body. Maybe this is the most important medicine.

I don't like bombastic statements from doctors about how long a person can survive. I believe it is impossible to say. Many of us have great confidence in authorities and are so thoroughly scared that we blindly believe in what the doctor tells us.

Our thoughts and feelings communicate directly with our body cells. If we accept a death judgment, the body may start to prepare itself to die. On the other hand, I have heard about and even met many who have reversed their doctor's judgment.

If a person chooses alternative treatment, it is very important to have the support of friends and family who believe in his or her choices.

There is a saying in Tibetan, "Tragedy should be utilized as a source of strength." No matter what sort of difficulties, how painful experience is, if we lose our hope, that's our real disaster.
—*Dalai Lama XIV*

Love and forgiveness

Anger, hate, fear, and a feeling of "poor me" are energies that often appear together with the cancer diagnoses. These emotions can literally eat you up from inside.

The most important part of my working through these feelings was forgiving those who have hurt me and reaching a deeper recognition of the belief that love, in fact, can solve everything.

I can see more and more that we all are doing our best.

Love and forgiveness have helped me to experience deeper inner peace and to have respect for all humans who have been involved in the painful dramas of my life.

Today I am good friends with my ex-husband, and we have a good collaboration regarding our kids.

It has also become clear to me that everything I have experienced as being tough and difficult to begin with has led me toward greater wisdom and made me a wiser woman.

Yes, crisis brings a great potential for us to grow and learn.

Love is the great miracle cure. Loving ourselves works miracles in our lives.
—*Louise L. Hay*

Exciting new acquaintance

In late summer 2002 I suddenly felt that I had drained out all my strength and was in need of a refilling. I signed up for a workshop weekend outside Oslo with a friend of mine. That Friday and Saturday became a great vitamin injection.

On Sunday we decided to gather some people who were open-minded. A man named Bent Madsen came to this session, and meeting him turned out to be a great experience for me.

Bent has been familiar with Dr. Hamer's research since 1989. He had searched for the secret of cancer for a long time, wondering what was lying behind all illnesses. He had both an engineer degree and had participated in numerous alternative therapy studies, but felt that something was missing. When Bent was reading an article about Dr. Hamer's research, he experienced a great "aha." He ordered the books of the German doctor, and two weeks later his first cancer patient consulted with him.

Meeting someone who was so interested in this exiting research was very inspiring for me.

Bent came from Denmark to Norway in 1989, and started up a wholesale business selling supplements and natural medicines.

When he discovered this research about the cancer riddle, he was inspired to share it with everyone who would listen. He was still into it and had shared this wisdom with many cancer patients during many years.

We really had something in common, and we also shared many other things, and a few weeks later we ended up as a couple.

What now, Dagfrid?

I was totally recovered and was finishing my art therapy education. I wanted to work as a therapist. *With my education and life experience, I thought, this is going to be easy.*

But things did not work out that easily, so I meditated upon the issue, and reached the following conclusion: I am going to work for the cancer issue.

I was led further along the way. My elder son moved in with me and helped me to establish my own website. This was an easy way to share information.

My history about computers is a bit funny. Computers scared me. My two small boys were utterly fascinated, and I was adamant: Never a computer for me! Later I learned "never say never."

When I became sick, I bought a computer and started to learn step by faltering step. The kids and my friends were considerately helpful and got me started. And now I am very happy about it. It is such a wonderful tool!

The very least you can do in your life is figure out what you hope for.
And the most you can do is live inside that hope.
Not admire it from a distance but live right in it, under its roof.
—Barbara Kingsolver, Animal Dreams

Help, I am invited to a TV show!

One beautiful afternoon in Bergen someone called me from the television show *Redaksjon 1*, a debate-show hosted by Viggo Johansen.

The show that evening was going to address the cancer issue and alternative medicine. Three doctors had accepted the invitation, and now they wanted a living example of an alternative-treated cancer patient.

Long ago I had decided never in my life to participate in a debate show. They follow a hectic tempo, and they rarely offer any in-depth elaboration. I was convinced of my conviction not to be in this setting, so my answer was a firm no.

The telephone rang again, and this time it was the host himself asking me to come. They had not been able to find anyone else who wanted to participate in the show. I became indecisive, because it was important for me to bring forth that idea people do have a choice about their treatment. I asked him for time to think it over. I took deep breaths. My heart and gut feeling said yes, even though my legs were literally shaking.

Three hours later I was sitting in the studio in Oslo. I was ready and totally calm.

I felt love toward the other participants in the show. All of us had our own truths, and the four of us had strong desires to share our truths. So we were not that far apart from each other really …

The debate became quick tempered, but the host had promised to take care of me—and he did. It felt strange sitting there together with three doctors who disagreed with what I had done to survive my cancer. Not one of them asked what I had done to get well or even showed any curiosity. I began to understand the deepest "truth" of academic medicine: Only the doctors can cure cancer.

I was amazed that neither politicians nor doctors are curious about how I saved the Norwegian state a fortune by just saying "no thanks" to their treatment. Though I do fully understand the lack of interest from the pharmacy industry.

I didn't interrupt or throw myself into the debate because that would have been like engaging in a kind of verbal warfare, and I didn't like that. The host gave me the opportunity to speak from time to time. The other debaters were stuck with their "truths" about why alternative medicines do not work. The patient's own contribution to healing is not anything the doctors were open to consider either.

During the show, viewers were encouraged to call in their answer to this question: "If you get seriously ill, would you consult alternative medicine practitioners?"

The answer on the screen was sensational: 85 percent answered yes.

Outside the studio I met the doctor who was supposed to be on "my side," because he was also using alternative treatments in his practice. On the air, though, he had said that if I had been his patient he would have recommended the removal my breast.

I asked him if he was familiar with the research of "the New medicine."

Yes, he said, in fact he was, but he was not going to study it seriously because he felt that if he did, he might be forced to forget everything he had learned.

That was a powerful finale for me. What a pity he had not had the courage to say that during the broadcast!

I felt so proud of myself. I had summoned the courage to be on a debate show, and I felt it had gone well. When I turned on my phone, there were thirty of forty massages from friends, all of them proud of me.

After the program I got a lot of letters and calls from people who had treated their cancer as I had treated mine, and they thanked me for coming forth.

We must believe that we are gifted for something, and
that this thing, at whatever cost, must be attained.
—*Marie Curie*

It's not always easy to share knowledge about this research

New challenges appeared.

When someone I knew well got a cancer diagnosis it was not always easy for me. Especially in the period just after I learned about Hamer's research.

I was very eager to make contact with these people and tell them about my own experience. I had a great wish to share everything I had learned.

Then I experienced something important. I realized it was very unethical for me to push this knowledge onto other people.

I really have learned to be patient.

I've learned to wait until the question is asked, because in the question lies the understanding of the answer.

Over the years I have learned that when someone asks I give them a "teaspoon" and not the whole "bathtub" at once.

Not everyone who experiences a shock will get cancer

It is important for me to emphasize this point: not everybody who experiences a shock will experience the development of cell abnormalities. It doesn't happen very often. Most conflicts get solved easily on their own.

The conflict or shock must meet four criteria before it can be called a "biological conflict shock":

1. The incident or shock occurs unexpectedly. It comes as a bolt from the blue.

2. The emotions caused by the incident are very strong.

3. Some of the emotions are so intimate that it is not possible to share them with others. The shock causes emotional isolation.

4. The person finds it hopeless to find a solution to the conflict.

The person experiences constant "thought buzz" about the event. It's the last thing he or she thinks about at night and the first thing he or she thinks of in the morning. It's like a video film that is playing all the time.

Most people have a great adaptability and find some solution that they can live with. This stops the cell changes, and the healing often goes unnoticed. These processes are natural

I believe that everything happens for a reason. People change so that you can learn to let go, things go wrong so that you appreciate them when they're right, you believe lies so you eventually learn to trust no one but yourself, and sometimes good things fall apart so better things can fall together.
—Marilyn Monroe

Cancer is often detected in the healing phase

In my studies I have come to a powerful new understanding as I have learned about the different bodily reactions during the phase of crisis (the cold phase) and the phase of healing (the warm, sweaty phase).

As humans we are wise souls and we are often able to find a solution to a conflict and release some of the deep emotional issues without professional assistance.

A lot of people I have met, read about, or heard about, who have been diagnosed with cancer, have already solved the initiating conflict and reached the healing phase.

In the healing phase they often feel deadly tired. They experience inner peace, lower blood pressure, fever, infections, and so on. Often people don't understand why they get sick, because emotionally they are feeling much better. This is when most people consult their doctors. They have not understood that something was wrong during the crisis. Maybe it is because we are so used to stress, problems, and a fast tempo of living.

There are so many interesting issues to think about.

The point of power is always in the present moment.
—*Louise L. Hay*

For cancer patients

Have you had experiences with radiation therapy, chemotherapy, hormone treatment, or surgery and are wondering if you did the right thing?

I feel that we all are doing the right things for ourselves. As long as we don't know about anything else we are choosing the right thing.

I find that it is very important to accept and feel at peace with the choices we have made.

We will always have new opportunities, and then we will understand the whole process in a different way and on a deeper level. The opportunity to get rid of old truths and replace them with something new is one of the gifts in this life.

It was wonderful to discover that I had the right to change doctors if the personal chemistry of one did not harmonize with mine. I have met several people who did the same and experienced the change as a pivotal point in the further development of their cancer story.

Don't be satisfied with stories, how things have gone with others.
Unfold your own myth.

—*Rumi*

Meeting a woman diagnosed with cancer

On that late summer afternoon when I met Bent, I also got to know Trine. She had been invited to our gathering in Oslo. We had talked on the phone earlier, and I invited her to attend our gathering. She had many exciting stories to tell.

A while ago she had felt a large lump in her right breast. She went to see her doctor who found it was cancer, and she knew that surgery and other treatments she had been offered were not right for her.

She contacted a man she knew who had an alternative understanding, and the next day she got the interview with Dr. Hamer on her doorstep.

Trine read it with care, gaining a deeper understanding about cancer. The ideas in the interview strengthened her decision to use only natural treatment. Trine had already experienced that synchronicities happened in her life.

In that same setting she also met Bent who was a thought field therapy (TFT) therapist.

A few days later, Bent was helping her to find the core issue of the cancer trauma. The emotions behind the conflict came to the surface.

The right coincidence at the right time.

Trine signed up for a class with Harald Baumann a month later, and when I told her about my own CT scan experience with Baumann, she got very excited and decided to have her brain scanned.

The interpretation of the images was significant both for Trine and her husband.

Harald Baumann confirmed that Trine had had cancer (he did not know anything about her on beforehand) and that she was in the healing phase. He prepared her for some bodily symptoms that she may experience. One was headache that occurs when the affected part of the brain begins to heal. That happened with Trine a while later.

It is much easier to go through symptoms and pains in the body when we know that they are a natural reaction and are caused by the body doing healing work!

I was excited to meet someone who was willing to go for a 100 percent natural treatment and who was looking at the cancer enigma the same way I did. We experienced enormous value in supporting each other on this nontraditional path.

After one year, the lump in Trine's breast was completely gone.

We were both delighted about the freedom it gave us to know about this groundbreaking research.

Today we are close friends, and both of us wish to spread the same message: Cancer is cell change caused by emotional conflicts.

The conflict needs to be dealt with, not pushed under the carpet.

I am full of hope that someday cancer research will open up and accept and embrace this knowledge.

Bent's adventure in God's laboratory

Ecology and taking care of nature has been my great engagement for many years. I have been actively involved in different environmental organizations through the years. When shopping for all of my groceries at health food stores, I have enjoyed trying to influence people, but I have not always succeeded.

When I met Bent it was an additional joy to become involved in his work with microorganisms. In the beginning of 1999 Bent was aware of EM—effective micro-organisms—in Denmark. This is a unique composition of microorganisms that participate in the ecological rebalancing of the soil where they are being used. Professor Teruo Higa from Japan developed EM more than twenty-five years ago.

Higa discovered that the microorganisms in the earth could be divided into three categories: vitality building, vitality disintegrating, and neutral.

EM consists of solely vitality-building microorganisms that are supporting each other. They are capable of rebuilding the perfect balance in humans, animals, plants, soil, and water. They are now being used in more than one hundred countries around the world.

Bent brought EM to Norway, and after further development and adaptation to Norwegian conditions, he introduced the product Vita Biosa. It was a great success and has helped many people cure a variety of ailments since then.

My ninety-year-old mama tried the product, and after using two and a half bottles of Vita Biosa she was very pleased. She had had diverticula on her colon for many years. After the treatment with Vita Biosa they were gone, and some other medical conditions too.

Even people with cancer have been helped, and I can recommend this treatment to everybody.

A companion product, Terra Biosa, consists of microorganisms for soil and plants. When I see how it is possible to grow healthy and tasty vegetables, grains, and fruits without using pesticides and inorganic fertilizers, my heart sings with joy. Now I know that someday in the future one of my wishes will come true: our society will be able to produce enough food for the entire population without polluting and exhausting our beautiful earth.

During the summer 2004 we took a trip around Scandinavia to film the results that gardeners and farmers were experiencing with Terra Biosa. What made the strongest impression on me was that animals that were given Terra Biosa were happier and healthier. It was a joyous trip.

I can fully understand when Bent announces that he is working in God's own laboratory where life is being created.

> *Everything you can imagine is real.*
> —*Pablo Picasso*

Fungi, bacteria, and viruses are our helpers

Research shows that a wide diversity of fungi, bacteria, and viruses are our good helpers when our health is recovering. It is proved how fungi and bacteria are able to break down and remove a lump of cancer when the initial emotional issue is solved. This is the healing phase.

These vitality-building microbes in the body carry an ancient memory that enables them to help the body heal itself. Knowing this has changed my attitude about my own bodily reactions.

When I have a cold, I know that I have solved a "stinking" conflict or a problem, and I congratulate myself on that. Then I curl up in bed feeling really good about it.

This knowledge has given me a great satisfaction. The body has a divine intelligence that allows microorganisms to carry out their wonderful functions.

Without knowing the cause of illness, any
treatment must be considered a guess.
—*Richard Diaz*

Exciting research on mammography

One day I discovered an article on the Internet news. It was an exciting read. The headline was: Breast Cancer Can Heal By Itself.

Two scientists, Jan Mæhlen, MD, PhD, professor of Pathology at Ullevaal University Hospital, and Per-Henrik Zahl, MD, PhD, medical doctor at The National Institute for Public Health, made this exciting discovery. They found that after mammography was introduced in both Norway and Sweden, there was a drastic increase in the number of diagnosed breast cancer cases, and there were more deaths after these checkups than there were before mammography was introduced.

They began to question. As many as two-thirds of women diagnosed with breast cancer after mammography have small tumors that would give no symptoms at all if they were left untreated. The mammography images often reveal small tumors, usually called benign tumors. These tumors would normally heal by themselves.

Too many women have been diagnosed with breast cancer because of the increasing use of mammography. The researchers claim that there is a connection between such over diagnosing and the new nationwide mammography examinations.

It is further revealed in their scientific report that, annually, about seven hundred Norwegian women are operated on unnecessarily.

Oh my God!

I called the researchers straight away, and I was told that their research was inspired when they wondered why their female colleagues did not examine their own breasts. Their work has made waves in the society of academic medicine, but also had drawn some attention from all over the world. It was published in several acknowledged journals.

I have, as I said before, had a mammogram once in my life, and it was just painful and nasty. Actually, I had the feeling that the test reduced and hurt my inner woman.

I have had those lumps that disappear too, and I have met many women who have told me the same story about lumps in their breasts.

Extensive studies are now being made in many countries on this relationship. One of the latest studies is from The Nordic Cochrane Centre. See the study on www.cochrane.dk. The Cochrane Collaboration is a network of more than thirty-one thousand researches from over 120 countries who work together to evaluate the effectiveness of health care practices.

Astounding research report on cancer

Else Egeland is a nurse and healer from Bergen. In 2004, she published her astonishing thesis. It contains interviews she had with eight people who had been diagnosed with "incurable" cancer disease, but who survived against all odds.

It is thrilling to read, and I can identify myself with their stories. We all did so many of the same things to recover!

The main essence was to encourage hope. Hope brings vitality, and maybe this is the main healer too.

Egeland recognized one common trait: all eight persons in her survey could relate their illness to life problems that they had experienced. They all chose to work with the circumstances in their life. They concentrated on strengthening the body and doing good things that also nourish the soul.

In two of the cases, the patients' doctors supported them after the patients were signed off as incurable patients. In the other cases, the doctors did not show any further interest.

Encouraging the self-healing powers is another common thread that runs through Egeland's wonderful thesis.

Her subjects chose different treatments in addition to being actively and positively involved with their cancer process. They all used a combination of several therapies.

Similarities between cancer patients who survived against all odds:

1. They decided to survive.

2. They thought: "Maybe there is something that the doctors don't know (yet)?"

3. They searched for new information to understand their sickness in a new way.

4. They gained new hope.

5. They used this hope actively, and hope led to action.

6. They seemed to be selective when they chose alternative treatment.

7. They called it "to do something myself" when they used alternative treatment.

8. They worked with all aspects of themselves, also at soul level and the existential.

9. They were active and disciplined—not passive about it.

10. They had people around them who were supportive and accepting their choices.

Else Egeland's main task
http://www.ub.uib.no/elpub/2004/h/122001/Hovedoppgave.pdf

My medicine chest

Many years ago I read Louise L. Hay's book *You Can Heal Your Life*. At the end of the book she provides a reference section. I have used this manual every time I have had a pain or illnesses in my body.

She refers to the possible emotional reasons for different diseases. This was my medicine chest for many years.

Later I was also been given the opportunity to expand this understanding of illnesses on a deeper level. I do thank Dr. Hamer, META-Medicine, Bent and my own experiences for this.

It is very valuable to learn about how the body reacts in two phases in a sickness. This applies not only to cancer, but to all diseases. This has urged me on to learn more about the inner healer. How valuable it is to listen to that inner voice and find out what feels right for me!

The human body is a unique creation, and it actually knows how to heal itself. This is an incredible gift that opens us up for even deeper understanding. We just need to arrange the right circumstances for it, either by processing the emotions involved or making some changes in our lives to solve our conflicts.

The body carries deep memories in those divine ancient cells that can tell the body what to do to obtain perfect health again. I understand that to fight against diseases is of no use. Indeed, fight only creates new fight, both within the body and the soul.

Modern academic medicine often uses the "killing" principle— against germs, viruses, and cancer cells. I can see that this only creates more imbalances. Media often perpetuate this idea with titles like "the war against cancer."

Doing things that are supportive to the self-healing process is more important than waging battles. I have always been fascinated by the traditional ancient remedies. I feel that modern medicine is very much founded in fear and financial gain. And so far it seems to me that many doctors do not want their patients to do anything for themselves.

I have never gone for my annual checkups. It has not felt right for me. I like knowing that I have the full privilege of deciding for myself whatever medical treatments I want to accept. It gives me a great feeling of freedom.

However, there have been times in my life when I have needed and benefitted from the help of academic medicine. I am glad they are there.

By disregarding intuition in favor of science, or science in favor of instincts, we limit ourselves.

Bernie S. Siegel

The joy of creating this book

It feels strange sitting here thirteen years after my cancer story and being able to share it with you. I never thought that I would ever get cancer, or that I would write a book. I am endlessly grateful that I had read Louise Hay's and Brandon Bay's books before I experienced cancer myself.

When you are in the midst of the crisis, the situation may feel insurmountable. The most important thing is to listen deeply to your own feelings for what is right for just you. Then you will get the support you need to go through exactly whatever it is that you need to experience.

It was no less than a miracle that I met an open-minded and non-judgmental doctor at Haukeland Hospital, and I was lucky to already have a holistic family doctor.

My stay at the ayurvedic clinic at Mesnalia contributed much in helping me gain the strength I needed to meet the challenge that came up at my follow-up checkup and the dramatic consultation with a young doctor. The gift was that I could take full responsibility for my own life.

The feeling of isolation is one symptom that cancer patients endure. The weekly telephone consultations with my deep psychology therapist were important in helping me to overcome this. And the two weeks I spent in his Health House were an added blessing. The people there, both staff and guests, gave me great gifts. They were brave souls who weren't afraid of cancer or deep and painful emotions. We all became close and helped each other.

Deep love from my children runs through the whole period like a red thread—and the wonderful unconditional love from my very special dog, Foxy.

It is so special to discover the "unplanned" yet related events that happen all the time. Synchronicity is one of life's magical gifts. These "coincidences" always carry messages in their wake.

Trust and hope have been reminders all the time ... letting go of that "good girl" who should always manage on her own.

I knew that I could not "fight against" cancer; rather, I had to collaborate so the healing could take place. I allowed myself to be a part of a whole, and I just knew that I would receive exactly the help that was necessary.

Today I am not afraid of cancer in general, and not afraid of what conventional medicine calls "spreading."

I fully understand how easily cell growth can be treated. It has taken me a long while to really let it sink in and to get rid of the former "truths" about cancer—and not only about cancer, but about other diseases too. I think it is a human right to have the opportunity to learn these things.

Yes, dear reader, I hope that you, who have been guided or inspired for some reason to read this book, will find something that gives you comfort or enthusiasm.

I understand well that you might still be full of questions, because I have presented new information about disease, and most of this information is not well known yet.

Personally, I have spent a great deal of time to change my be-lief systems. It has been both frustrating and confusing at times. I understand if you maybe feel frustration? Or maybe you recognize something that has been your truth for some time?

For many years I have known that I had to come forward with my story. It has taken some time to reconstruct the story because it was important for me to put the difficulties behind and live as much as possible in joy and the now moment. This new way of thinking has resulted in many great gifts. Now I feel ready, and I am writing in great joy.

As I write, I am filled to the brim with deep gratitude and happiness for everything that I have learned. I realize that I have grown and have become a more balanced and a wiser human. My ability to love has grown stronger, and I have met so many wonderful people. I am very happy about all I was able to learn.

Please keep in mind that this was my path, and these were my choices. There are as many roads to Rome as there are people. I got to know cancer from my own body; that was my road. My personal growth has benefited enormously from this experience.

I am so happy to write my story; my heart will be warmed if people find inspiration and hope by reading it.

I want to give thanks to all of you who supported me in different ways along this path. And a special thank you to my dear Bent, who has been my closest source of inspiration.

His deep knowledge of Hamer's research, META-Medicine, integrative medicine and modern epigenetic along with his own experience in trauma treatment, has been a great inspiration for me.

During the years after I had met Bent, we have together spent years to better understand what cancer and other diseases really are. We both have a big thank you to all the open minded doctors, scientists and therapists who have inspired us on this journey.

It is a great pleasure for me to be able to share some of this knowledge with you dear reader.

My background

I was born on a farm on the west coast of Norway in 1954. I was the sixth girl in a family of seven siblings. From my earliest childhood I learned to work like the boy my parents always hoped to get.

At the age of fifteen, I met the man who became my life partner for thirty-one years. He lived by the same beliefs that I did: work hard and be very good at it.

I began as an exhibition decorator in retail stores, a creative profession that gave me a lot of wonderful challenges.

My husband took over his father's electrical installation business in steps, and he expanded further.

We worked more … and more … and we enjoyed it in a way, because of the satisfaction of being busy and feeling that we were useful.

Even after our two sons were born, it was not enough for me to just be a mother for them. We had children in foster care too.

This "being good" pattern followed me even after I became interested in natural healing.

I always had several projects going on, and my calendar was full. Something had to happen all the time—kids, friends, workshops, books, and philosophizing …

This was an informative and exciting period.

Crises can appear as gifts to us. They make it possible for us to stop in our tracks and look inside and ask, What do I feel? It was wonderful to discover that my crisis actually brought me great gifts.

My philosophy is to "view life as a mirror." If I attract something that hurts, it's the old "wounds" from my childhood that might be given the opportunity to be transformed.

Today I can see it was my great lack of inner self-esteem that created my pattern of being a "good girl." I thought I needed to achieve and show others that I was good enough. I did not believe that I deserved to be loved for just being me. Maybe someone recognized this?

And this conception is not easily turned around in a flash. It was quite a distance to walk to get rid of these feelings.

Accepting and loving myself followed in the wake of this process. It has taken time. I now enjoy more and more the simple joy of being alive!

When we expand our thinking and beliefs our love flows freely. When we contract we shut ourselves off. Can you remember the last time when you were in love? Your heart went ahhh!! It was such a wonderful feeling. It is the same with loving yourself except that you will never leave once you have your love for yourself. It's with you for the rest of your life, so you want to make it the best relationship that you can have.
—Louise L. Hay

From teacher to farmer

In 2006 Bent and I were led further on to International META-Medicine Association (IMMA), an international network of open-minded people having the same basic views on the mind-body connection that Dr. Hamer has, but they have included and integrated the latest research from epigenetic, trauma treatment and many other research branches. It also includes the principle of love, spirituality and the gift we humans can receive when we have lived through a crisis and a disease in our life. META-Medicine is today regarded as the spearhead in integrative medicine. We joined the network, and have since been teachers in this wonderful knowledge of META-Medicine as approved master trainers.

For more information about META-Medicine:
www.metamedicine.info and www.metahealthuniversity.com

This teaching has given us many wonderful years meeting open-minded people. And we have really felt the pleasure of teaching many people to understand how shocks, conflicts, emotions, and disease are related.

We started seminars and training in Norway, and were subsequently invited to Estonia and Denmark. We taught for many years, until there were others who were ready to take over the sharing of this knowledge.

In Norway there was an abrupt end to our teaching when we experienced a bullying campaign in the media against us in 2009. It was a big shock that drove us into a deep crisis, but we worked our way through our reactions and came forth unto the gift of this life experience.

I had been longing to live on a farm again, and now it was time to look for the perfect place. Finally it popped up in a strange way, and we were "farmers" again. This has been very important, especially for me.

I love having free-range animals around me, and I love living in a silence that is free from all manmade noise. I love to hear the beautiful sounds of nature, to hear the sounds of the river both in drought and abundant rain, to hear the rooster that crows when people are coming or when his hen flock is threatened by a hawk or a fox.

I love to hear the wind and storm, thunder and lightning, plants and animals ... they all speak to us.

My heart sings with joy when I hear the ringing of the bells that our sheep wear around their necks. They are always near the house. In fact, they are our living lawnmowers, because our beloved farm is so steep that we can't cut the grass.

Self-sufficiency has been important for both Bent and me, and we experience a great pleasure by growing our own organic vegetables. Bent has continued to produce Biosa microorganisms which we use to drink, give to our animals and use in the garden and greenhouse.

When we were building our greenhouse, we felt like kings of the hill ... happiness beyond all happiness.

I feel ready to share my cancer experiences with the English-speaking world. It is a story that I hope might inspire others who find themselves in similar situations.

> *How wonderful it is that nobody need wait a single*
> *moment before starting to improve the world.*
>
> *—Anne Frank*

Bent Madsen's background

Bent was born 1945 in Denmark, where he obtained a degree in engineering. After some years, his interest in the "alternative" world of medicine was so great that he changed his profession and became a therapist, specializing in classical Chinese acupuncture.

He moved to Norway in 1989. When his daughter was diagnosed with type-1 diabetes, he promised her and himself that he would spend all the time he needed to find the true cause of diabetes.

He was jubilant when he discovered Hamer's research in 1989 and finally understood the cause of type 1 diabetes. He knew at once, in both soul and mind, that this theory felt right. His engineering training enabled him to recognize immediately that it was the voice of truly natural laws.

In the following years he completed a number of courses in nutrition, homeopathy, Reiki healing, thought field therapy (TFT), neuro-linguistic programming (NLP), and more.

In 1999 Bent began to develop Biosa microorganisms inspired by the Japanese researcher Dr. Teruo Higa. Bent's dream was to give all Norwegian farmers and gardeners the opportunity to produce organic crops without reduction in crop yields. He succeeded in proving it.

It turned out that the Norwegian society was not yet ready for these changes. There were huge financial interests in retaining the current system.

Once again he turned his main interest to understand disease at a deeper level. He spent all of his time to investigate many sources to really understand the mind–body connection. Along with Dagfrid he created manuals and the directory that were used in the upcoming seminars and workshops.

For some years Bent has been master trainer in META–Medicine. Together with Dagfrid he has traveled in Norway, Denmark, and Estonia to hold seminars and train others in this wonderful knowledge.

Part II

The META-Medicine model of the disease process

Bent Madsen

Introduction

META-Medicine is not a therapy or treatment, and it does not involve diagnoses in the traditional way. META-Medicine is a scientific framework for understanding how life experiences, emotions, and reactions in the body are interrelated. It is a model that has shown an amazing accuracy in practice.

META-Medicine gives people the opportunity to understand the causes of their own disease processes, how to be healed, and how to prevent diseases. We have very often observed that, when a person has become aware of the real cause of his or her illness, then a healing process can begin automatically.

Many events in daily life can be experienced as a tsunami.

In our modern society, we can often feel powerless when something unexpected happens. We feel that we are not in control of our own life situations. We may feel ashamed, we may be afraid of hurting others, we might worry about being alone, or we might stress over economic concerns. The list is endless, and is different for every person.

Here is a list of the types of daily-life conflicts and traumas that can cause biological shock:

- Divorce or breakup of a relationship, or the fear of this happening

- Being dismissed from work, or the fear of this happening

- Being bullied at school or the workplace

- Being physically or psychologically abused

- Experiencing fear in connection with a medical diagnosis

- Death of a loved one, or fear of separation

- Surgery or anesthesia.

Of course there are many more.

It is important to state that it is not these happenings in and of themselves that are the cause of further medical problems. It is the individual person's own reaction and subjective emotional experience that is at the core of resulting disease. Additionally, what one person experiences as a shock will not necessarily affect others in the same way.

The natural life processes

In all living organisms, from human beings down to the amoebae, the life processes can be understood as a constant condition of rhythmic exchange between expansion and contraction: During the day, the sympathetic nervous system dominates and puts us in a positive state of stress, so we have the energy to cope with the challenges that life gives us. At night, the parasympathetic nervous system dominates, so we can exhale and relax, and we can recharge the "batteries" again.

During the course of evolution, nature has developed optimally appropriate responses to dangerous situations for all organisms. This is to ensure the survival of the individual and the species in the most optimal way.

In an unexpected and dangerous situation, the natural day-night rhythmic cycle is put on hold. The entire organism instinctively and instantaneously goes into a state of alert preparedness. Here the sympathetic nervous system rules. When the situation is resolved, there is a shorter or longer period where the individual "breathes out" in order to get back to the normal state. During this period the parasympathetic nervous system dominates.

The disease process from stress phase to healing phase

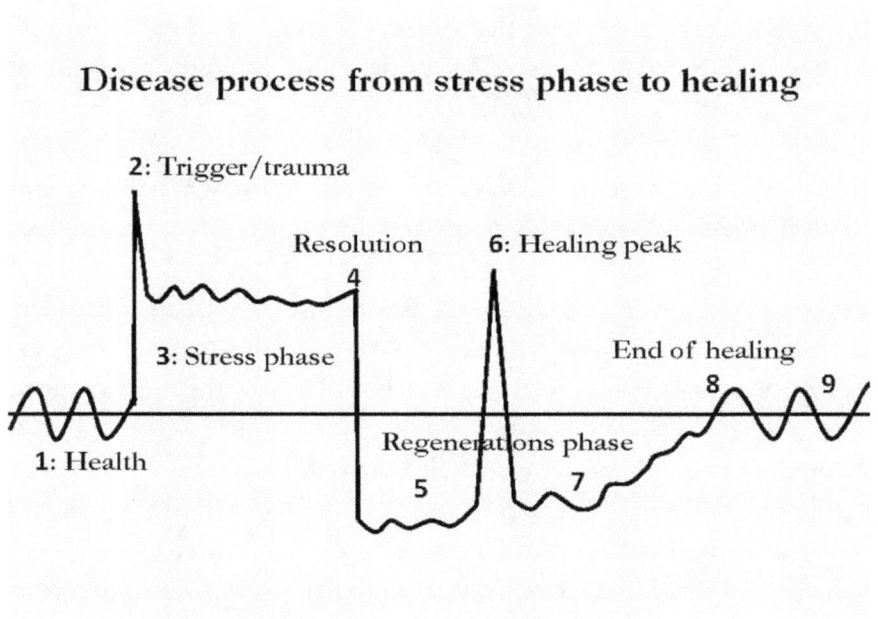

Disease process from stress phase to healing

2: Trigger/trauma

Resolution
4

6: Healing peak

3: Stress phase

End of healing
8   9

1: Health

Regenerations phase
5   7

Following is a point-by-point explanation of the disease process:

Point 1: Normal health

This is "normal life" experienced by a rhythmic exchange between activity during the day and rest at night.

Point 2: A conflict shock or trigger occurs

This is experienced as an intense emotional incident, which hits suddenly and unexpectedly. We are caught unawares. It strikes like lightning. Finding a solution seems hopeless. We have no strategy.

In that very moment of conflict the hormonal status of the body is altered, and the organism is put on red alert.

Instantaneously and simultaneously the emotions, the brain, and the body and organs are affected.

It is important to emphasize that, at the very moment the "lightning" strikes our personality is altered. Our perception of our environment as well as our reactions are affected.

In META-Medicine we always seek to ascertain what the patient thought and felt during the seconds in which the conflict manifested.

Once a pattern is impressed on the brain, disease will automatically correspond to it. Unless we become aware of this "track," triggers can automatically cause relapses, which will follow the same pattern.

Point 3: The stress phase, also called the cold phase

When it is impossible to find a solution to the conflict, we are kept locked in the cold or frozen phase where the sympathetic nervous system overrides all reactions.

The conflict, or stress, phase is characterized by the following symptoms:

- Continuous stressful thinking about the problem.

- Believing that a solution is hopeless.

- Cold hands and feet, as well as poor appetite, which can lead to weight loss. This happens because the blood supply to the muscles gets priority.

- The blood supply to the frontal lobes decreases to the advantage of the more primitive part of the brain.

- Cold sweats and pale skin may occur.

- The conflict contains elements and emotions that are so intimate that it is difficult to share them with anyone. One withdraws.

- There is an increase of stress hormones such as adrenaline, cortisone, and others. This often leads to muscular tension.

- Sleep problems may occur causing a person to often wake up shortly after having fallen asleep.

- An increase in blood pressure and pulse may occur together with heart palpitations.

- An increase of glucose in the blood may occur.

- Dryness of eyes and mouth frequently occurs.

- The breathing pattern is affected. One holds one's breath or breathes in a more shallow and rapid manner.

- There may be cell alterations or functional disturbances, depending on which part of the brain the conflict corresponds to.

All processes in the conflict phase have biological significance and aid in pushing the individual to find a solution to the conflict.

Point 4: Conflict solution

When a solution to the conflict is achieved, the development of the stress phase stops and the organism enters a healing phase. Often life offers practical solutions to conflicts and traumas. For instance, someone has lost a partner meets a new one, or a person finds a new job after having been unemployed, or gets a new puppy after a treasured dog has been run over by a car.

In other cases, the conflict may be solved on the emotional, mental, or spiritual level.

Point 5: *The first part of the healing phase: the warm phase*

After a solution to a conflict occurs, there is a corresponding change in the entire organism. The state of alert is shut off, and the parasympathetic nervous system becomes dominant once again. It is often in this first phase of the healing that we really feel ill.

If there has been cell growth in the conflict phase, this will now be decomposed by fungi or bacteria in the healing phase. If there has been cell shrinkage in the conflict phase, there will now be a repair through cell growth in the healing phase.

The first part of a healing phase is often called "the sweaty phase."

This phase is characterized by the following symptoms:

• There is peace of mind. One may finally relax.

• Blood supply returns to hands and feet, which now become warm.

• There may be warm perspiration often with raised temperature. Fevers, inflammations, and infections may occur. One may feel sick and go to the doctor.

• There may be a great need to talk about what has been happening and to share it with others. One opens up to the world and to life.

• There may be a period with an enormous (at times death-like) fatigue.

• There may be better quality of sleep and a need for more sleep.

- Blood pressure and pulse are normalized. There may be periods with low blood pressure and slow pulse.

- There may be clear eyes and plenty of saliva.

Point 6: Healing peak

If the conflict has been intense and prolonged, a healing peak may occur when the relaxation is at its highest. Sometimes it may cause problems, with symptoms; for instance, cramps, epileptic seizures, double vision, dizziness, fainting, headaches, or migraines among others. Simultaneously, at a certain point in this phase, a short-term revival of conflict emotions can occur; the person may feel that the conflict is suddenly active once more.

Point 7: Urinating phase

When the healing peak is over, the last part of the healing phase occurs, in which all surplus water is excreted. Slowly and imperceptibly our days get better and better, and one day we discover to our amazement that we feel 100 percent well; we are full of vigor and vitality.

Point 8: Normal health

The process of the disease has now been completed and we are back to normal health.

Point 9: Attaining awareness

Perhaps the most important point in a disease process is attaining a greater awareness.

- How was this perfect for me?

- What did I learn?

- How has my insight grown through this experience?

- How can I arrange my life in order to avoid illness in the future?

- What is of real value to me?

The fundamental principle of evolution seems to be that all beings can develop only through encountering changes, trauma, and other challenges and then choosing to learn from them. This is how the individual grows in knowledge and wisdom and is raised to the next level of self-development.

Escaping emotional isolation

The conflict moment—the moment the lightning strikes—is often stored in memory as a fourteen-second "video" that runs over and over again, causing constant "thought buzz." This little "movie short" often contains all the information about the emotions necessary to process to start the healing phase.

Some of the emotions are so intimate that we find it impossible to share them with others. There may be emotions of shame, anger, inadequacy, and more, and emotions that may be perceived as unethical, immoral, or condemned by the environment or oneself.

The main thing is to get out of this emotional isolation and share with others. It can happen with a therapist, a psychologist, a mentor, or close friends. This single step may sometimes be sufficient to stop further cell growth.

Transformation of emotions

When we are coming out of the emotional isolation, the next step is to process all the bad feelings. Epigenetics is the study of how factors other than DNA sequence can control genetics. Research has shown that our strongest beliefs, feelings, and thoughts directly affect and program how our genes are expressed. In this way, our emotions affect the biological response of our cells, our hormone balances, and how our immune system works.

We always have options in how we react to an event.

In an extreme negative reaction, we maintain a feelings of rage and hate. We refuse to forgive. This makes us feel like a victim; we harbor feelings that the event is unfair.

In an extreme positive reaction, we understand and integrate the underlying causes of our own actions and the actions of others who may be involved. Then we understand that we are all doing the best we can; we remind ourselves that everyone, in early childhood, has been imprinted with individual belief systems. We understand that it is these beliefs that unconsciously govern our behavior. This awareness can lead to total forgiveness of oneself and others. In this way, the bad feelings from the event may disappear like snow in spring.

When the painful emotions are transformed in a positive way, the self-healing powers are initiated, and the body automatically goes into a healing process in which the hormone balance is restored.

Meanwhile, we have a unique opportunity to learn to know ourselves. This is often the start of a wonderful self-developmental process.

For most people, it can be very valuable to seek the help of another person when trying to understand this process. It is best to find a person or a therapist whose "chemistry" fits. It should be someone who has insight into these relationships and also has masters the techniques that can be used to release repressed emotions.

Many therapists currently have knowledge of "energy psychology" and explore it through neurolinguistic programming (NLP), thought field therapy (TFT), emotionally freedom therapy (EFT), eye movement desensitization and reprocessing therapy (EMDR), and others. These therapeutic methods can often produce rapid and sustained results, especially if the therapist also has knowledge of META-Medicine.

At the very moment the emotional isolation is broken and emotions are transformed, hormone status changes and cell growth stops. The body goes from defense mode to repair mode.

New understanding about cancer spreading?

This new psychosomatic understanding shows us that conflict shocks, emotions, and traumatic events usually are the triggering factors in disease.

It is a known fact that a diagnosis of a serious disease can often cause new emotional shocks and conflict situations. For example, if a patient experiences an existential conflict in connection with a grave primary diagnosis, this conflict can become the triggering factor for a cell alteration in the liver. Here the emotion "afraid of starving to death" has its organ-related location.

The feeling may be quite literal, provided the body is unable to absorb sufficient nutrition during a chemotherapy cure, intestinal surgery, or treatment with morphine.

It may also be figurative; for example, a fear concerning one's economy during the period of illness.

Additionally, it may be a more general anxiety about one's existence.

Cancer of the liver is rarely the primary diagnose in rich countries; more often it is the second or third diagnose. In the poorest countries in the world, however, liver cancer is the dominating primary form of cancer, caused by a fear of literally starving to death.

We find the same conditions related to lymph nodes and the skeletal system. These are the organ-related location of various self-worth conflicts. Similarly, cell alteration in the lungs can be caused by fear of death.

Through mapping of countless patient cases it has been shown that proliferation of cancer in the body generally follows the individual emotional experiences of shock. It can often occur in the wake of a cancer diagnosis. Therefore we might ask ourselves whether it is the hypothesis of aggressive cancerous cells that proliferate, or is it new emotional experiences of shock that is the most common reason for proliferation?

Our experience is that patients who choose to include META-Medicine in their program of treatment lose their fear of proliferation. They are more attentive to the importance of processing the emotions that might arise, and frequently get through the period of treatment with fewer side effects and more peace of mind.

Part III

Excerpts of the directory of mind–body connection

Bent Madsen

Introduction

The following list of common diseases and the reasons behind them has been built over many years. The starting point was back in 1989 with the research of Dr. Hamer. Over the years it has been complemented, extended and developed further by my own research, by studies of the academic medicine and psychology and by investigating the last decade multidisciplinary research which scientifically proves that all life experience, from the very good to the extremely painful, is reflected both in the brain, in the nervous, endocrine and immune systems and "inward" in the cells in which the genetic material DNA is regulated and activated. It is also inspired from meetings with hundreds of clients and meetings with numerous workshop participants.

The list in this book is an excerpt of the mind–body directory and is in short form. It is my hope to release a complete directory sometime in the future

Excerpts from the mind-body directory

Altered voice: see Larynx

Anemia: see Bones

Appendix: appendicitis

Type of conflict:

This is a conflict that is perceived as ugly, indigestible anger.

Example: a child overhears his or her parents quarrelling and fighting. It cannot be "digested"; it is "repulsive."

Conflict phase:

In the conflict phase there is either a secretory compact cell growth, which may close the appendix, or flat resorptive cell growths that "thickens" the cell walls.

Healing phase:

After the conflict has been resolved, an acute or semi acute appendicitis occurs when the cell growth disintegrates through fungi or bacteria.

Arteriosclerosis: see Blood vessels

Arthritis: see Bones

Blackheads: see Skin

Bladder I: bladder inflammation, blood in the urine

Type of conflict:

This conflict is perceived as ugly, repulsive, threatening, or troublesome ... something nasty.

Examples: A pregnant woman is beaten by her husband. A person experiences a strong psychic pressure.

Conflict phase:

In the conflict phase there is a compact secretory cell growth or there are smaller resorptive polyps.

Healing phase:

After the conflict has been resolved, the cell growth disintegrates through virus or bacteria, which can cause bladder inflammation.

Bladder II: mucous membrane, blood in the urine, bladder inflammation

Type of conflict:

Man: The conflict is related to masculine territorial markings for the purpose of defining a position.

Woman: The conflict is related to feminine territorial markings for the purpose of establishing a border within one's own territory: who decides in the home.

Conflict phase:

In the conflict phase there is cell necrosis in the bladder mucosa.

Healing phase:

After the conflict has been resolved, the ulcers may bleed. There may be pain and cramps and some swelling. It may be difficult to urinate even though the pressure is great. After a while the condition is normalized.

Bladder III: sphincter muscle: incontinence, bed-wetting

Type of conflict:

There is a territorial marking conflict; someone invades the person's territory.

There is an inability to define limits. The person's identity is violated.

Conflict phase:

In the conflict phase there is cell necrosis in the striated muscles of the bladder wall. This may cause the sphincter muscle to become relaxed to the extent that incontinence follows.

Healing phase:

After the conflict has been resolved, the muscles are rebuilt and the sphincter muscle functions again.

Blood in the stool: see Intestine

Blood in the urine: see Bladder I and Bladder II

Blood sugar, low: see Pancreas alpha cells

Blood vessels, arteries: arteriosclerosis, high blood pressure

Type of conflict:

This is a self-devaluation or disability conflict in which the contents of the conflict relate to specific areas of the body (see Bones).

In the conflict phase there is heightened blood pressure and more rapid pulse.

Conflict phase:

In the conflict phase there is cell necrosis in the inner wall of the artery. The walls of the arteries can become so thin that they rupture, and this can give rise to a collection of bruises or bleeding. The plaque cells that have been torn off may completely block the artery and cause thrombosis.

Healing phase:

After the conflict has been resolved, repair takes place, and the necrosis is filled with plaque. With each conflict increasingly thicker layers are built up, and the condition becomes arteriosclerosis.

Blood vessels, veins: varicose veins, phlebitis

Type of conflict:

This is a self-devaluation or inferiority conflict in which the contents of the conflict relate to specific areas of the body (see Bones).

It often involves the feet, in which case the conflict can be a feeling of someone or something being a hindrance (the person feels he or she is "dragging a ball and chain").

Conflict phase:

In the conflict phase there is cell necrosis in the inner wall of the veins involved.

If the feet are involved, there may be cramps.

Healing phase:

In the healing phase, wounds form to repair the cell shrinkage. This provides a swelling of the vein wall and surrounding tissue. After several periods of conflict and solutions, the characteristic varicose veins develop.

Bones: anemia, leukemia, osteoporosis, arthritis

Type of conflict:

This is a deep self-devaluation and inferiority conflict in which the affected area mirrors the problem. It is a conflict that "goes to bone and marrow," and it stems mostly from comparing oneself with other people's expectations or self expectations.

Skull and neck vertebrae: The topic is mainly intellectual, such as injustice, disharmony, morality, and coercion.

Jawbone: The conflict is an inability to speak one's mind in a quarrel or disagreement.

Right shoulder/arm: This is a mother/child/home conflict in a left-side-dominant person, and partner/father conflict in a right-side-dominant person. This conflict is an inability to hold on.

Left shoulder/arm: The reverse of the right shoulder/arm.

Spine: This is a conflict of personal self-devaluation and inferiority.

Lumbar region: This is a central personal self-worth conflict, and it affects entire personality.

Ribcage: Self-devaluation. For instance after having had a breast removed, or after surgery on heart or lung.

Breastbone: Self-devaluation. For instance after heart- or other surgery.

Hip/femoral neck: This conflict arises from an inability to tolerate a situation … an inability to break through a resistance. To be stuck.

Pelvic area: This conflict is related to sexuality and gender.

Knee: This conflict is about feelings of not being fast enough; for instance in connection with sport. Also, feelings of being inflexible and being stuck in a situation.

Ankles and feet: For instance, in connection with dancing. This conflict arises from not able to run away from something, from being inflexible. It reflects a lack of equilibrium.

Hand: This conflict is about being unable to tackle or do something, or being unable to hold on.

Conflict phase:

In the conflict phase there is a contraction of the blood vessel and a decalcifying of the skeleton. There is a decrease in the forming of red blood cells, as the bone marrow may also be involved. This can cause anemia.

The periosteum is intact and keeps the structure in place almost like a kind of bandage. Spontaneous fractures are rarely experience during this phase.

Healing phase:

After the conflict has been resolved, the bone swells and the periosteum expands. This can be very painful, and there is a risk of spontaneous fractures. The calcium returns and rebuilds the knuckle.

Immediately after the solving of the conflict, the entire blood circulatory system expands in order to better direct nutrition into the affected bone areas. The total amount of blood fluid increases correspondingly. The contents of all kinds of blood cells per milliliter of blood fluid is therefore altered. In the beginning this looks like an acute anemia. Simultaneously there is an extreme increase in the production of white blood cells, which in the beginning don't reach maturity. This is diagnosed as leukemia. After four to six weeks, the production of red blood cells also gets underway, and slowly the blood values are normalized.

If the decalcification has been near a joint, arthritis may develop where the liquid calcium is being squeezed out at the joints.

Breast mammary glands

Type of conflict:

Right breast:

For a right-hand-dominant person, this is a conflict over worry, argument, or fight with partner, colleague, boss, or father.

For a left-hand-dominant person, this is a conflict over worry, argument, or fight, mostly with child, mother, or home, or nest.

Left breast:

Reverse of the right breast.

Conflict phase:

There is a proliferation of the glands cells, which can be diagnosed as a benign fibro adenoma or as a lobular breast cancer.

Healing phase:

After the conflict has been resolved, the cell proliferation immediately stops, and the tumor either becomes encapsulated or disintegrates. A slight swelling accompanied by some pain may occur during the disintegration. At the end of the healing phase, there may be some pain as the tissue shrinks and forms scar tissue.

Breast intraductal: retracted nipples, reduced breast size

Type of conflict:

Right breast:

For a right-hand-dominant person, this is a conflict of separation or fear of separation from partner (also father, boss, colleague, friend, grown-up child, and so on).

For a left-hand-dominant person, this is a conflict of separation or fear of separation from children or something perceived as a "child." Also from one's mother, home, or nest.

Left breast: reverse of the right breast.

Conflict phase:

In the conflict phase there is cell loss in the mammary ducts. This causes an ulcerative dilation and a slight tension and only minimal pain, and is seldom discovered. In a conflict of long duration, the breast can become increasingly hollow, and the nipple can become completely retracted. The skin may have reduced sensitivity.

Healing phase:

After the conflict has been resolved, the cell shrinkage stops and a rebuilding repair starts. The mucous membranes around the ulcers swell. This may cause formation of "lumps" that in the building phase can be diagnosed as benign growths, as carcinoma in situ, or as a malignant carcinoma of the mammary ducts. The breast may swell and become red. Often there is an increased sensitivity and some pain. After the healing is complete, the breast may be smaller and harder.

Cavities: see Tooth enamel

Colic: see Intestine

Colitis: see Intestine

Common cold: sinusitis, nosebleeds

Type of conflict:

This is a "stinking conflict." The entire situation stinks, almost always figuratively speaking.

This reflects something that is worries about ... something that gets on the nerves.

This is something to be sniffed at, to have a hunch about ... something about which danger or another problem is suspected.

The goal is to get rid of the stench (the worry).

Often, a person in a stressful job situation catches a cold when he or she goes on a vacation. It is a temporary solution for getting away from everything that causes the stress.

Conflict phase:

In the conflict phase there is cell loss in the mucous membranes of the nose and/or the sinuses.

If the sinuses are involved there may be pain.

If only the nose is involved, there are only rarely symptoms. The nose may possibly feel dry.

Healing phase:

After the conflict has been resolved, the mucous membranes swell, with or without bacteria. Fluid is plentiful (runny nose). The nose may get extra sensitive, become itchy, and feel slightly painful.

If the sinuses are involved they will now be less sensitive and without pain.

Constipation: see Intestine

Crohn's disease: see Intestine

Diabetes type I: see Pancreas beta cells

Ear: hearing loss, tinnitus

Type of conflict:

This is caused by not wanting to hear something: "I can't believe my ears." It could be caused by an unexpected and emotional communication on the telephone. It is very often related to either people or territory.

Tinnitus may result from triggers—secondary warning signals to avoid the same or similar situations.

Conflict phase:

In the conflict phase there is cell loss with reduced hearing at certain frequencies. Tinnitus may occur.

Healing phase:

After the conflict has been resolved, the inner ear swells during repair and may give a temporary deafness. Later the hearing function returns to normal.

Ear, middle ear: middle ear infection

Type of conflict:

Right ear: This conflict arises from a disability to believe in something, and perhaps a need to hear specific information. It can also reflect a fear of missing out on something.

Left ear: This conflict arises from an inability to let go of something one has heard (can't get it out of one's head).

Conflict phase:

In the conflict phase there is resorptive cell growth in the middle ear.

Healing phase:

After the conflict has been resolved, decomposition through fungi or mycobacteria takes place. This causes a puss-filled inflammation or even a perforation of the eardrum during the healing crisis. Later it returns to normal.

Eczema: see Skin

Emphysema: see Lung alveoli

Esophagus mucous membrane, upper 2/3 of esophagus

Type of conflict:

This is a conflict over not wanting to swallow (accept) or digest a fact, thing or happening, but feeling forced to do so … wanting to spit it out again.

It is a conflict over wanting to rid oneself of something.

Conflict phase:

In the conflict phase there is cell loss with the forming of ulcers. This can give cramps and pain when swallowing food.

Healing phase:

After the conflict is resolved, there is an intense swelling of the ulcer and minor problems when swallowing. There may also be bleeding. It is often at this stage that the diagnosis of a narrowed esophagus is made. The condition rectifies itself after a while.

Esophagus, lower 1/3 of esophagus: hernia, heartburn

Type of conflict:

This is a conflict over being unable to swallow the outcome of an issue about a wished-for thing or happening. Often this concerns a car or a house or similar goal that the person wants but suddenly cannot have.

This condition brings feelings of "this is unfair" or "if it had only been like this …"

Conflict phase:

During the conflict phase either a compact secretory cell growth is formed, or there are many small resorptive cell growths.

Healing phase:

After the conflict has been resolved, the cell growth sponta-neously dissolves, either by fungi or mycobacteria. This may cause a strong smell. Often this growth is not diagnosed but disappears on its own.

Eye, retina, nearsightedness, farsightedness

Type of conflict:

This is conflict over a fear of some danger or threat from behind. Something or someone is threatening or lurking from behind and cannot be shaken off. It is a fear of something one cannot do anything about—a disease, loss of job, a test, and so forth.

Nearsighted: This reflects a fear of one's surroundings and a subsequent withdrawing into oneself. The person thinks ahead with anxiety and uncertainty. It may involve a fundamental fear in connection with survival, trust, and security in life.

Farsighted: In this conflict, the attention is turned outward in order to avoid looking at one's own issues. The facade is more important than who one really is. Anger is suppressed for fear of hurting others. This causes the person to react to a threatening world by focusing outward and not letting things affect the self. This person thinks of the past with anger, self-justification, or with a sense of not having done the right thing.

Conflict phase:

In the conflict phase there is a reduced functioning of parts of the retina.

This may be different in the two eyes. The vision may decrease on parts of the eye or on the entire eye.

Healing phase:

After the conflict has been resolved, an edema forms between the synovial membrane (sclera) and the retina which altars the shape of the eyeball. When the edema is gone, the vision may return to normal.

If we get a "hanging healing phase" in which the conflict is repeatedly triggered and resolved, calcification between the synovial membrane and the retina forms, maintaining the abnormal shape of the eyeball.

In nearsightedness, the eyeball is optically stretched and stays that way because of the calcification.

In farsightedness, the eyeball is optically pressed together and stays that way because of the calcification.

Facial paralysis

Type of conflict:

This conflict is caused by a feeling of losing face, being made fun of, a fear of being tricked or cheated. This person can't "keep up the mask." There are thoughts of "What will they think of me now?" "I can't see them now, as they laugh at me."

Conflict phase:

During the conflict phase the function of the facial muscles is lost. It's not the muscles but the nerve signals that control them and become reduced or completely blocked.

Healing phase:

After the conflict has been resolved, the functioning returns to normal. At the height of healing there may be painless spasms in the muscles.

Fibromyalgia

Type of the conflict:

This is a conflict of self-devaluation, often concerning one's looks and/or ambitions. It is a syndrome that affects muscles, tendons, and connective tissue.

Conflict phase:

In the conflict phase, there is cell loss (atrophy) of the involved muscles, connective tissue, and tendons. Symptoms may include fatigue with light tension and a little pain.

Healing phase:

After the conflict has been resolved, muscles and tendons are reformed.

If a hanging healing phase develops, it is diagnosed as fibromyalgia. The symptoms are pain and reduced mobility.

Fungal mouth infection: see Mouth and palate

Gall colic: see Liver ducts

Gastritis: see Stomach

Goiter: see Thyroid gland

Hemorrhages: see Uterus, cervix

Hemorrhoids: see Rectum

Heartburn: see Esophagus

Hepatitis: see Liver ducts

Hernia: see Esophagus

High blood pressure: see Blood vessels

Hyperthyroidism: see Thyroid gland

Hypothyroidism: see Thyroid ducts

Incontinence: see Bladder III

Intestine I, smooth muscles: colic, constipation

    Type of conflict:

For the first part of the intestine, the conflict arises over the inability to accept a matter, object, happening, or emotion.

For the central part of the intestine, the conflict arises over the inability to get ahead with a matter, object, happening, or emotion.

For the last part of the intestine, the conflict arises over the inability to let go of a matter, object, happening, or emotion.

Conflict phase:

There is locally increased peristalsis (to push the "piece" further) and reduced peristalsis in the rest of the intestine. Symptoms may be constipation.

Healing phase:

After the conflict has been resolved, peristalsis of the intestines is increased. This usually causes digestive discomfort and colic before the condition gradually becomes normal.

Intestine II, colon: ulcerative colitis, air in the intestine, blood in the stool

Type of conflict:

This conflict results from ugly, indigestible anger or bitterness.

Example: Being falsely accused of having tried to betray someone. A woman discovering her husband is having an affair with her best friend.

The conflict brings feelings of "This is making me sick." "I cannot accept this."

If the affected area is in the ascending colon, the conflict is with close family members.

If it is in the transverse or descending part, more periphery people are involved.

If it is the lower part of the colon (sigmoid) that is affected, conflict elements of nasty, dirty feelings cannot be jettisoned.

Conflict phase:

In the conflict phase either a compact secretory cell growth forms and may become so large that it blocks the passage in the intestine (produces gastric juices), or there are smaller resorptive cell growths that thicken the intestinal wall. Often there is an increased production of gastric acid. Other symptoms include digestive discomfort, weight loss, alternating constipation and diarrhea. The condition can also be without symptoms.

Healing phase:

After the conflict has been resolved, the cell growth decomposes through fungi or mycobacteria with or without bleeding. During this phase it may cause night sweats that culminate in the morning.

The intestinal disease known as ulcerative colitis is a "hanging healing phase" in which the conflict is repeatedly triggered and followed by a solution. Symptoms may include diarrhea with blood and mucus, painful bowel movements, poor appetite, abdominal pain, and fever.

Intestine III, small intestine: Crohn's disease

Type of conflict:

If the upper part of small intestine is affected: the conflict is an inability to digest a certain "matter" or anger, and often involves an additional aspect of a "hunger" for something.

If the lower part of small intestine is affected: the conflict is an inability to digest a certain "matter," often connected to fear of being hungry in the broadest sense; for instance, going bankrupt.

Conflict phase:

In the conflict phase there is a cell growth of flat cells (cells with only a few layers), which rarely causes intestinal blockage. The cell growth secretes in order to increase the capacity for digestion.

Healing phase:

After the conflict has been resolved, the cell growth decomposes through fungi or bacteria. This often leads to bleeding. This can cause temporary digestive discomfort with blood and mucus in the stool before the condition becomes normal.

The intestinal inflammation disease Crohn's disease is a "hanging healing phase" in which the conflict is repeatedly triggered and followed by a solution. Symptoms may be an inflammatory condition with bleeding, diarrhea, abdominal pain, nausea, weight loss, lethargy, and mild fever.

Jaundice: see Liver ducts

Kidney collecting tubules: kidney inflammation, "refugee conflict"

Type of conflict:

This is a conflict of existence and/or abandonment and/or isolation—not feeling at home ... the experience of losing everything, or feeling totally exhausted: "My life is falling apart."

This brings feelings of isolation and helplessness, feeling entirely alone, not feeling taken care of, feeling as if one is being treated badly ... "wandering in the desert." This is a common feeling during hospitalization.

Conflict phase:

In the conflict phase either a compact secretory cell growth forms or smaller resorptive cell growths form. The body retains water, which can cause edema or an increase in weight. In rare cases, urine poisoning and kidney failure result.

Healing phase:

After the conflict has been resolved, there is an encapsulating or a bacterial dissolving of the cell growth, and after a phase marked by frequent urinating, the condition normalizes.

Kidney renal pelvis mucosa: kidney stone, renal colic

Type of conflict:

This is usually a territory marking conflict. It can be masculine or feminine. It has to do with establishing a border within one's own territory: "I failed to make my mark."

Conflict phase:

In the conflict phase there is cell loss (ulcers) to make room for a greater stream of urine. This may cause light cramps with only slight pain.

Healing phase:

After the conflict has been resolved, repair occurs that can cause swelling, pain, and kidney cramps (colic). The pains culminate when the kidney stones are pressed out into the renal pelvis. After this the cramps cease and the kidney stones pass down into the bladder and out of the body.

Larynx mucous membrane: altered voice, vocal cords

Type of conflict:

This is a conflict of shock and fear when a completely unexpected danger threatens. It can cause an inability to speak because of fear, and paralysis and not knowing what to say. It can also be a territorial fear conflict in which the danger appears imminent. Often it concerns a neighboring house, a job, a business, a partner, a strife, and more. The conflict arrives like a lightning strike.

Conflict phase:

In the conflict phase there is cell loss with ulcers in the throat and/or the vocal cords. There may be light pain or light voice alteration and some difficulty in speaking.

Healing phase:

After the conflict has been resolved, repair causes a great swelling of the area. This can result in a great alteration of the voice, because polyps may form on the vocal cords. Symptoms may be increased sensitivity with "tickling" in the throat, dyspnea (difficulty in breathing), and chronic hoarseness.

Leukaemia: see Bones

Liver (parenchyma)

Type of conflict:

This is a fear of starvation conflict—an existential conflict. It can be for oneself or for others.

Examples: Fear of not being able to manage financially due to illness. Fear of bankruptcy. Fear of losing one's means of existence.

It can also be a biological hunger conflict when the body is unable to get sufficient nutrition because of intestinal illness, an eating disorder, chemotherapy, or famine.

Conflict phase:

In the conflict phase there is cell growth in the liver. This can be secretory or resorptive. It is a single round focus when the conflict concerns other people, and multiple when conflict concerns oneself.

Healing phase:

After the conflict has been resolved, the cell growth can become encapsulated and the liver can form new substitution tissue. The liver may swell a great deal, and fatigue and night sweats may be experienced.

Liver ducts, bile ducts: gall colic, jaundice, hepatitis

Type of conflict:

This is a conflict of anger relating to territory. Often it concerns money or a neighbor, a rival, or a colleague who oversteps his or her limits. This conflict brings feelings of "This is my domain." "I have failed to uphold my duty."

Conflict phase:

In the conflict phase there is cell loss in the ducts of the liver and/or gallbladder, which may cause moderate pain, colic, or the vomiting of bile.

Healing phase:

After the conflict has been resolved, there is repair in the form of cell growth. The first sign is increased cholesterol and bile. This may, over a short period, result in jaundice when the bile ducts are blocked because of strong swelling of the mucous membranes.

The healing may also appear as hepatitis A or B, or hepatitis non-A or non-B, depending on what virus the body has at its disposal with which to try to complete the healing.

Lung alveoli: emphysema, tuberculosis

Type of the conflict:

This is usually a matter of an unconscious or conscious fear of death; for instance, following a cancer diagnosis, accident, or during wartime. It may also be a fear of someone else dying.

Conflict phase:

Immediately following the conflict, a cell growth of small resorptive tumors begins. The growth continues until the conflict is solved. There are single small growths when the fear concerns someone else, and many, perhaps connected, small tumors when the fear concerns oneself. The diagnosis goes from a benign lung alveoli tumor up to a malignant lung carcinoma.

Healing phase:

After the conflict has been resolved, the growth stops and the tumors often become encapsulated. If tubercle bacillus are present, they will begin to decompose the tumors and will leave cavities in the lungs after the healing is completed. There may be night sweats, coughing, and vomiting of blood. Tuberculosis is thus a healing symptom following lung cancer.

If many alveoli are destroyed during the process of healing, emphysema may result as a symptom.

Lungs bronchial mucous membrane and muscle: bronchitis, pneumonia

Type of conflict:

This is a conflict of fear about territory. The opponent has not yet attacked, but the danger seems imminent. It may also be fear that someone will leave one's territory without permission.

Conflict phase:

In the conflict phase there is cell loss in the mucous membrane of the bronchi in order to make room for a greater intake of air. Mucous membranes lose their sensitivity. The condition is rarely discovered.

Healing phase:

After the conflict has been resolved, there is cell proliferation to reform the mucous membranes. They swell and may become overly sensitive. The swelling may cause insufficient air supply to the small alveoli, which can make breathing difficult.

The condition is often diagnosed as cancer of the bronchi.

A frequently occurring symptom is a cough that may last for months. During the healing process, this may turn into pneumonia. If the bronchial muscle also has been involved there may be violent convulsions during the healing peak, and this is diagnosed as bronchitis.

Lymph

Type of conflict:

This conflict arises from light self-devaluation. It affects the lymph nodes and vessels corresponding to the skeleton area (see Bones). Emotions and worries in connection with a cancer diagnosis often have an effect on the lymph nodes in the throat area.

Conflict phase:

In the conflict phase there is cell loss, which forms "holes"; lymph nodes viewed in a microscope may resemble Swiss cheese.

Healing phase:

After the conflict has been resolved, the lymph nodes swell, and the holes are filled with cell growth. The diagnosis is often malignant lymph tumors.

Melanoma: see Skin

Menstrual cycle, irregular: see Ovaries

Middle ear infection: see Ear

Mouth and palate deep-seated mucous membrane: fungal infection, mouth ulcers

Type of conflict:

Palate:

Right side: Conflict arises when a person obtains a wished-for thing, but is unable to "swallow" it. (For example, a person believes he has won the lottery, but finds out that the ticket was not handed in.)

Left side: Conflict arises when a person is unable to "spit out" something … cannot get rid of something … wants to spit something out.

Mouth:

Right side: Conflict arises when a person is unable to get hold of something. (For example, a sick person cannot take in food because of pain.)

Left side: Conflict arises when a person is unable to rid oneself of something or someone.

Conflict phase:

In the conflict phase there is either secretory or resorptive cell growth.

Healing phase:

After the conflict has been resolved, fungi or mycobacteria decompose the cell growth. There may be a strong smell during the decomposition, or it may be diagnosed as a fungal infection.

Mouth ulcers may also occur; these usually do not cause any symptoms.

Mouth and tongue mucous membrane: mouth ulcers and ulcers on tongue

Type of conflict:

Mouth: This conflict is about not being able or willing to take something into the mouth. An example is a driver who has to breathe into an alcoholmeter, knowing he will lose his driving license.

Tongue: This conflict is about not being able or willing to put something into words. It is about being without language, being unable or afraid to simply "spit out" what one really means.

Conflict phase:

In the conflict phase there is cell loss with the forming of ulcers in the mucous membranes of the oral cavity or the tongue. This can be very painful.

Healing phase:

After the conflict has been resolved, there is an intense swelling of the mucous membranes during the repairs, often accompanied by bleeding. After three to six weeks, there is only a slight scarring left.

Mumps: see Parotid gland

Muscular paralysis, multiple sclerosis, and Parkinson's disease

Type of conflict:

This is a conflict of self-devaluation with regard to "mobility."

When it occurs in the feet, it is an inability to flee or follow, or an inability to decide whether to come or go or a feeling of being stuck in a situation.

When it occurs in the arms and hands, it is an inability to hold on, or to defend oneself.

When it occurs in the shoulders and back, it is an inability to escape.

The conflict always involves an element of being trapped in the situation (see Bones).

The biological meaning is to "play dead," as the situation appears hopeless.

Conflict phase:

In the conflict phase there is a progressive paralysis related to the intensity of the conflict. Few or no nerve impulses from the brain centers in question reach the involved parts of the body. Single muscles or entire limbs may be affected. The condition is not painful but may give rise to other emotional trauma.

Healing phase:

After the conflict has been resolved, edema is formed in the affected areas of the brain. At first it looks as if this is causing a further reduction of the muscular functioning and is accompanied by uncontrollable shaking. As healing continues, the brain edema recedes and is followed by a slow healing in which the functioning gets better and better.

Often we see the conflict is not completely resolved, and the patient experiences repeated small relapses. This also often happens in dreams. It prevents the healing from ever reaching completion. Such a "hanging healing phase" is diagnosed as Parkinson's disease.

The actual diagnosis "you have multiple sclerosis and will never be able to walk normally again" contributes to maintain and strengthen the suffering. The patient must realize that the disease *is* curable, and that others have succeeded.

Myoma: see Uterus muscle

Nosebleeds: see Common cold

Osteoporosis: see Bones

Ovaries I: inflammation of the ovaries

Type of conflict:

This is a conflict of strong emotional loss or separation from children, husband, best friend, parent or pet.

Conflict phase:

A compact secretory cell growth (teratoma) forms. This can cause an increased level of estrogen.

Healing phase:

After the conflict has been resolved, the cell growth slowly stops. Like other embryonic tissue, it has a built-in period of growth. Mycobacteria can dissolve the cell growth before the condition is normalized.

Ovaries II: irregular menstrual cycle

Type of conflict:

A conflict of inconsolable loss resulting from death or emotional separation from children, husband, parent, best friend, or pet, or something perceived as "my child."

Conflict phase:

In the conflict phase cell decomposition occurs; it is normally not detected. Estrogen levels are often low and can cause irregular menstruation.

Healing phase:

After the conflict has been resolved, the necrosis are refilled. One or more cysts form, slowly being filled with connective tissue. This is often diagnosed as ovarian cancer, as the cyst attaches itself to near organs in order to ensure blood supply for its growth. After nine months, the cyst becomes a firmer lump (is indurated) and detaches itself from other organs. The cyst produces extra sex hormones, but can be removed if it causes problems.

Pancreas alpha islet cells: low blood sugar levels

Type of conflict:

This conflict is centered around fear and disgust in connection with someone or something specific.

Examples: Being forced to eat or drink something disgusting. Rats. Stinking thrash. Something nauseating. Also a lack of sweetness in life.

Conflict phase:

In the conflict phase there is an increasing loss of functioning in the alpha cells of the pancreas, causing deficient ability to produce glucagon. This leads to increased levels of insulin followed by low levels of blood sugar.

Healing phase:

After the conflict has been resolved, there is a slow normalizing of the blood sugar levels. There may be periods of unstable high and low blood sugar levels.

Pancreas beta islet cells: diabetes type 1

Type of conflict:

This conflict involves resistance and defense against someone or against something specific. It is to bristle against someone or something, or to struggle against someone or something.

Conflict phase:

In the conflict phase there is an increasing loss of functioning in the beta cells of the pancreas, causing deficient production of insulin and increased blood sugar levels.

Healing phase:

After the conflict has been resolved, the blood sugar level slowly sinks. There may be insulin-producing cell growth. There may be periods of unstable high and low blood sugar levels, especially in the healing peak.

Pancreas: inflammation of the pancreas

Type of conflict:

This is often a family conflict in which one fights over something one wants. There are struggles over things and quarrels with other people. There is much anger.

Example: Conflicts over the settlement of inheritance.

Conflict phase:

One or more secretory cell growths in the pancreas forms. This causes an increased production of pancreatic juice, which may cause nausea and loss of appetite, resulting in weight loss.

Healing phase:

After the conflict has been resolved, the cell growths may either become encapsulated or disintegrate, leaving cavities in the gland. Following this the condition is normalized.

Parkinson's disease: see Muscular paralysis

Parotid gland secretory ducts: mumps

Type of conflict:

This conflict arises over an inability to eat—one does not want to eat, is not allowed to eat, or feel forced to eat (usually figuratively, to accept something or someone). It is a conflict of having something forced onto one.

Conflict phase:

In the conflict phase there is cell loss with ulcers in the secretory ducts (makes room for increased secretion of saliva). The area becomes extra sensitive and may cause slight dragging pain.

Healing phase:

After the conflict has been resolved, the ulcers are repaired with or without viruses. There is a swelling that blocks the secretory ducts. This causes the well-known swollen condition that is so characteristic of mumps.

Periosteum: rheumatism, numbness of skin

Type of conflict:

There exists a brutal conflict of separation resulting from a pain we have caused someone, or that someone has caused us. (The pain can be real, but it is usually an emotional experience.)

Conflict phase:

In the conflict phase there is a functional reduction in the periosteum. The connected network of nerves becomes supersensitive and causes fleeting stabbing pains (rheumatic pains.) The area corresponds to the area in which we have been hurt or where we have hurt others.

Healing phase:

After the conflict has been resolved, the function is re-established. Now there is reduced nerve sensitivity, except in a healing peak when the pains may reoccur and sometimes last one to two weeks. Other pain during this phase is caused by the healing of a self-devaluation or inferiority conflict that has affected the knucklebone itself.

Phlebitis: see Blood vessels

Pimples: see Skin

Pneumonia: see Lungs bronchial

Polyps: see Throat

Prostate

Type of conflict:

This is a gender conflict that is experienced as nasty, scary, threatening, troublesome, or ugly.

Examples: An elderly man left by his younger girl friend who moves in with a younger man. Not being master in one's own home. Not feeling sufficiently manly. Often it can be an ongoing conflict—worry over a lessening vitality, or inner uncertainty about one's value as a man. It can also be caused by changes in the relationship between a man and a woman, or changes in the reaction pattern of partner after menopause.

Conflict phase:

In the conflict phase a secretory cell proliferation is formed and causes increased production of secretion, thus a greater volume of seminal fluid.

In rare cases the cell growth may press on the urethra and make it difficult to completely empty the bladder. By far the majority of men beyond the age of forty-five to fifty have an enlarged prostate and live out their lives without serious problems with the condition.

Healing phase:

After the conflict has been resolved, the cell growth stops and there is an encapsulating or decomposition of the growth (an inflammation), after which the condition is normalized.

Psoriasis

Type of conflict:

This is a conflict of separation—a sudden loss of physical contact with parents, partner, friend, pet, and so forth. It also is the opposite: too much unwanted and unavoidable contact.

The area involved reveals the topic of the conflict. If it is the right arm, it often has to do with the partner. If it is the inside of the elbow, it has to do with wanting to hold onto someone; if it is on the outside of the elbow, it has to do with wanting to keep someone at a distance.

Conflict phase:

In the conflict phase there is often insufficient blood supply, which causes reduced sensitivity, hardening of the outer layer of skin, and sometimes peeling.

Healing phase:

After the conflict has been resolved, the skin becomes red and warm when the blood supply increases and new cells form. There is increased sensitivity.

A special point is that active conflict can continually alternate with the solution to the problem. An example is a child who does not want to be separated from the mother but must every day in order to attend kindergarten.

Rashes: see Skin

Rectum: hemorrhoids, boils

Type of conflict:

This conflict involves an unpleasant, ugly, outrageous, or disgusting accusations that are perceived as deceitful, mean, or evil. This is usually in connection with people in one's immediate family or vicinity. It fosters feelings of not being able to let go ... a "dirty" conflict ... not being able to let go of one's rage.

Conflict phase:

In the conflict phase flat resorptive cell growths or more compact secretory cell growths are formed. These can cause difficult passage or complete closure.

If they are located higher up, they are growing underneath the mucous membrane and can be felt but not seen.

Healing phase:

After the conflict has been resolved, the cell growth disintegrates, accompanied by light bleeding and perhaps night sweats.

If the cell growth is underneath the mucous membrane, boils may form, resulting in hemorrhoids. Following this the condition is normalized.

Rectum mucous membrane: bleeding hemorrhoids

Type of conflict:

This is a feminine conflict of identity that causes feelings of not knowing where one belongs, where one ought to be, where one should go, or what one should decide to do.

Conflict phase:

In the conflict phase there is cell ulceration of the rectum, allowing more excrement to mark one's position (identity).

Healing phase:

After the conflict has been resolved, there is a painful swelling of the mucous membrane. There may be bleeding, and the condition is often diagnosed as bleeding hemorrhoids.

Rectum sphincter muscle: involuntary bowel movement

Type of conflict:

This is a conflict of territorial markings. A person's area is invaded; he or she is unable to define limits.

Conflict phase:

In the conflict phase there is cell necrosis of the striated muscles of rectum. This causes the sphincter muscle to become relaxed, open, and leak.

Healing phase:

After the conflict has been resolved, the muscles are rebuilt and the sphincter muscle functions again. At the height of healing there may be a passing reoccurrence of the leakage.

Reduced breast size: see Breast

Refugee conflict: see Kidney

Renal colic: see Kidney

Retracted nipples: see Breast

Rheumatism: see Periosteum

Shingles: see Skin

Sinusitis: see Common cold

Skin (dermis), pimples, blackheads, shingles, melanoma

Type of conflict:

Dermis:

This conflict is brought on by a feeling of being dirty ... a violation of one's integrity ... a feeling of being deformed (for instance after an operation). Also, figuratively, it is like being called a "dirty pig."

Shingles:

The conflict arises from a feeling of being dirty or of having dirt thrown at one ... a feeling of discomfort in an embrace ... a feeling of being "disfigured" (for instance after a breast operation).

Sweat glands and sebaceous glands:

Forehead: This conflict arises from light intellectual self-devaluation, for instance in connection with school.

Neck: This conflict arises from a feeling of being talked about behind one's back.

Face and chest: This conflict arises from uncertainty over encounters with other people.

Conflict phase:

In the conflict phase there is cell growth in order to strengthen the skin layer and provide better protection.

Dermis: If birthmarks are involved, a compact melanoma with pigmentation forms; otherwise, skin cancer without discoloring forms. There is no pain.

Shingles: Small points of cell growth are formed underneath the upper layer of skin. The points may congregate so that they form larger or smaller segments. There is no pain.

Sweat glands and sebaceous glands: Small compact cell growths are formed. There is no pain.

Healing phase:

Dermis: After the conflict is resolved, the cell growth stops and decomposition with mycobacteria or other bacteria takes place.

Shingles: This is a nerve infection caused by a reactivating of dormant chickenpox virus. The healing phase can be very painful. If the upper skin layer breaks open, there is a strong smell.

Sweat glands: During the decomposition, typical ripe pimples form, which can be squeezed out.

Sebaceous glands: During the decomposition, the familiar blackheads form. There is no pain.

Skin (epidermis): eczema, rashes

Type of conflict:

This is usually a matter of sudden loss of physical contact with parents, partner, children, family, pets, and so on.

It may also be the opposite—not wanting contact with someone or something.

The location of the skin problems can often reveal the contents of the conflict:

For right-hand-dominant people, the right side is the partner side, and the left side is the parent/child side. For left-hand-dominant people it is the other way round.

If it is on the inside (for instance the inner side of the elbow) it signals a wish to hold on to the contact. If it is on the outside, it may be a wish to keep someone at a distance. If it covers large areas of the body, it is a major central conflict of separation.

Conflict phase:

In the outermost layer of the skin there is a poor supply of blood and microscopic sores with cell loss form. Sensitivity is reduced, and the skin becomes rough and dry. Finally the skin may peel.

Healing phase:

After the conflict has been resolved, there is an increase of the blood supply, and the microscopic rash is healed. The skin becomes red, warm, and slightly swollen and may itch. This phase is called eczema or dermatitis. If there is a repeated reactivating of the conflict, or only a partial solution, the condition may remain; it becomes "chronic."

If the conflict and its triggers are resolved, the skin can often be fully healed in the course of a few days.

Stomach and duodenum: heartburn, gastritis

Type of conflict:

This conflict is caused by an inability to digest something, a quarrel with family members, an inability to get one's rightful share. It often concerns money, inheritance, or a court case.

When the duodenum reacts, the conflict is often quarrel or anger in connection with family members, in the workplace, or with friends, and so on.

Conflict phase:

In the conflict phase either a secretory cell growth develops that can become as large as a head of cabbage, or a smaller resorptive cell growth develops (thickening of the stomach wall).

These can cause increased production of stomach acid and acid regurgitation (heartburn).

Healing phase:

After the conflict has been resolved, fungi or bacteria decompose the cell growth, or an encapsulating occurs. The amount of acid becomes normal.

Inflammation or ulcers (gastritis) may occur for a period before the healing is completed.

Stomach and duodenum mucous membrane: ulcers

Type of conflict:

This is a biological reaction to a territorial conflict that incites anger; for instance, a conflict with neighbors. It can also be a conflict within one's territory, such as a partner who is unfaithful, gambles, or causes other problems.

Conflict phase:

In the conflict phase there is cell loss in the mucous membranes of the stomach's small curvature and especially around the mouth of the stomach, or in the duodenum. Ulcers form and may cause pain, cramps, and colic.

Healing phase:

After the conflict has been resolved, there are bleeding ulcers with black feces, but without pain and colic. Vomiting may occur.

Teeth dentin:, gum inflammation, inflammation in roots of teeth, loose teeth

Type of conflict:

This is a self-devaluation conflict ... a "biting-conflict" ... a feeling of being unable to bite back or not having the heart to bite back, or not having the strength to defend oneself. It can be the result of being bullied at school, at work, at home, and so forth.

If it occurs in the corner teeth, it is a feeling of being too weak to catch something or to hold onto something or someone.

If it occurs in the front teeth, it is a feeling of being too weak to bite back or bare one's teeth.

141

If it occurs in the cheek teeth, it is a feeling of being unable to grind or process something or someone.

Conflict phase:

In the conflict phase there is cell shrinkage that causes the formation of holes in the inner part of the tooth, underneath the enamel. The holes can be seen in X-rays. With repeated or strong conflicts, the jawbone is also affected and the tooth can loosen. As the tooth may now be wriggled, it leads to the neck of the tooth becoming exposed.

Healing phase:

After the conflict has been resolved, the calcium returns to re-build the tooth and the jawbone. This is the phase when there will be swelling and possibly toothache. Other symptoms may be bleeding gums and inflammation of the root of the tooth.

Teeth enamel: cavities

Type of conflict:

This is a self-devaluation conflict caused by feelings that one is not allowed to bite back. It causes one to have a defensive attitude. "If he were not my boss, I'd tell him what I really think."

If it occurs in the corner teeth, it is a feeling of not being allowed to grab hold of or hang onto something or someone.

If it occurs in the front teeth, it is a feeling of not being allowed to bite back or bare one's teeth.

If it occurs in the cheek teeth, it is a feeling of not being allowed to grind or process something or someone.

Conflict phase:

In the conflict phase cavities—tooth decay—are formed in the enamel. This may cause extra sensitivity and pain in the tooth.

Healing phase:

After the conflict has been resolved, the enamel slowly re-forms without pain but with sensitivity to heat, cold, sweet, or sour.

Testicle I

Type of conflict:

This conflict is caused by profound loss by death or emotional separation from children, wife, best friend, parent or pet.

Same content of conflict also often manifests in the lymph nodes around the lumbar vertebrae.

Conflict phase:

A compact secretory cell growth (teratoma) is formed. This may result in an increased level of testosterone.

Healing phase:

After the conflict has been resolved, the cell growth slowly stops. Like other embryonic tissue, it has a built-in period of growth. Mycobacteria may decompose the tumor. After this the condition is normalized.

Testicle II

Type of conflict:

This conflict arises after profound loss by death or emotional separation from children, wife, best friend parent or pet

The same type of conflict also often manifests in the lymph nodes around the lumbar vertebrae.

Conflict phase:

In the conflict phase there is a cell loss with necrosis, which is normally not noticed. Testosterone level may decrease.

Healing phase:

After the conflict has been resolved, the cell shrinkage stops and the scrotum swells. A cyst forms which gradually fills up with connective tissue, which produces testosterone (increasing the chances of new offspring). Unless this is physically bothersome, it does not cause problems and can be tolerated for the rest of one's life.

Testicle III, bi-testicle: inflammation

Type of conflict:

This is a conflict of territorial competition, territorial fear, or territorial loss. Often it has a sexual element regarding the partner.

Conflict phase:

In the conflict phase there is cell loss in the mucous membrane of the bi-testicle.

Healing phase:

After the conflict has been resolved, there is reparatory cell growth with swelling of the mucous membrane, which can lead to painful inflammation before the condition becomes normal.

Throat: polyps

Type of conflict:

This is a conflict about not being able to get hold of or hang onto something.

Conflict phase:

In the conflict phase secretory polyps grow, increasing the ability to "swallow" something more rapidly.

Healing phase:

The polyps decompose by means of fungi or mycobacteria. There may be a strong smell during this phase.

Thyroid gland: hyperthyroidism, hard goiter

Type of conflict:

Right side: The conflict is over an inability to get hold of something, or an inability to manage in a competitive situation because one is not quick enough to get what one wants.

Left side: The conflict arises because one is not quick enough to get rid of someone or something.

If the affected organ is the bi-thyroid gland:

Right side: The conflict is over an inability to "swallow" something, a fact, or an experience (muscles have reduced ability to contract due to lack of calcium).

Left side: The conflict is over an inability to "spit out" something, a fact, or an experience.

Conflict phase:

In the conflict phase there is cell growth with the formation of a compact secretory tumor. The cell growth gives increased production of thyroxin and thus increased metabolism in order to make the individual faster (for example, enable the person to solve the crisis). This is called a hard goiter or struma.

Bi-thyroid gland: Only the secretory type can increase the calcium level in order to increase the muscular contractions.

Healing phase:

After the conflict has been resolved, the cell growth may dissolve by means of bacteria, and the hormonal balance will then be normalized. Often the cell growth becomes encapsulated, and then there is a continued slightly raised hormonal level.

Thyroid glandular ducts: hypothyroidism

Type of conflict:

This is a conflict over a feeling of being powerless: "Something must be done urgently, but my hands are tied and nobody does anything." "I cannot change the situation." "I want to be in control."

Conflict phase:

In the conflict phase there is cell loss with ulcers in the glandular ducts. It cannot be seen, but can sometimes be felt when it causes tension.

Healing phase:

After the conflict has been resolved, there is a swelling during the repair. In some cases a cyst forms, which fills up with connective tissue. This is termed benign goiter or euthyroid struma.

During the swelling, the outflow of thyroxin may temporarily be reduced. By repeated occurrences this can cause scar tissue so that the condition becomes "permanent," and cause low metabolism or hypothyroidism.

Tinnitus: see Ear

Tonsils: tonsillitis

Type of conflict:

Right side: This is a conflict over being unable to "swallow" something or not getting something or someone that one badly wants.

Left side: This is a conflict over being unable to "spit out" something or someone … being unable to get rid of something.

Conflict phase:

In the conflict phase there is a secretory cell growth in order to increase secretion. This enlarges the tonsils, and they may look inflamed, but there are usually no problems.

Healing phase:

After the conflict has been resolved, fungi or mycobacteria decompose the surplus tissue, followed by characteristic tonsillitis with discharge of pus.

Tuberculosis: see Lungs alveoli

Uterus cervix, uterine mouth: lack of menstruation, hemorrhages

Type of conflict:

This is usually a sexual conflict or a sexual frustration conflict that is connected to not being able to mate (become pregnant). It is a deeply instinctive drive. It can be caused by separation from the partner. If the woman uses contraceptives, the body may still react with frustration over not becoming pregnant.

The conflict can also derive from the opposite: One ought not to mate. In addition, there can be an unconscious guilty conscience if one has many sex partners.

Conflict phase:

In the conflict phase there is cell loss (ulcers) at the mouth or neck of uterus. Often ovulation stops and menstruation does not occur. The ability to achieve vaginal orgasm is often lost.

Healing phase:

After the conflict has been resolved, viruses form repair tissue in order to make up for the cell shrinkage.

There may be bleeding from uterus or cervix. This phase is usually diagnosed as cell alteration in the cervix (cervical-carcinoma or portio-carcinoma). Menstruation starts again.

Uterus mucous membrane: strong bleeding

Type of conflict:

This may be a femininity conflict concerning one's feminine sense of honor. It can derive from receiving comments such as "You are a bad mother," "Yu are a boring sex partner," or "You behave like a man."

It can also be a conflict of loss; a grandmother/grandchild conflict; or an unpleasant, partially gender-specific conflict with a man.

Conflict phase:

In the conflict phase either a compact secretory cell growth or several small resorptive cell growths form in the mucous membrane in the uterine cavity (adenocarcinoma).

Healing phase:

After the conflict has been resolved, the tumors are excreted together with the mucous membrane of the uterus during strong bleeding.

If the woman has reached menopause, it will decompose more slowly, with discharge and moderate bleeding before final healing (Fluor vaginalis).

Uterus muscle: myoma

Type of conflict:

This is a conflict of self-devaluation connected to not being able to carry through a pregnancy. Figuratively, it can be doubt about one's ability to carry through a wish, a "fetus," an idea, or future dream and see it through to "delivery." It can stem from an unfulfilled longing to have children or not being able to hold on to penis (hold on to a man).

Conflict phase:

In the conflict phase there is cell growth that makes the muscle stronger. One or more myoma may optionally be formed.

Healing phase:

After the conflict has been resolved, there is cell loss. If there is a myoma it can now be broken down and excreted, or it may stay until menopause when it diminishes by itself.

Varicose veins: see Blood vessels

Vocal cords: see Larynx

Bibliography

Bays, Brandon. *The Journey: A Practical Guide to Healing Your Life and Setting Yourself Free*. New York, Atria Paperback, 2012.

Billander, Susanne. *META-Health: Consciously Healing Body and Soul*. Amazon, 2013.

Bourbeau, Lise. *Your Body's Telling You: Love Yourself!. The most complete book on metaphysical causes of illnesses & diseases*. Stockholm, Vattumannens forlag, 2008.

Edwards, Gill. *Conscious Medicine: Creating Health and Well-Being in a Conscious Universe*. London, Hachette Digital, 2010.

Fisslinger, Johannes R. *META-Health—Decoding your body's intelligence*. Los Angeles, Meta-Health University, 2013.

Flook, Richard. *Why am I sick? How to Find Out What's Really Wrong Using Advanced Clearing Energetics*. London, Hay House Ltd., 2013.

Hamer, Ryke Geerd. *Scientific Chart of Germanic New Medicine*. Alhaurin el Grande, Spain, Amici di Dirk, 2007.

Hay, Louise L. *You Can Heal Your Life*. Santa Monica, Hay House, 1984.

Lee, John. R., M.D., David Zava, Ph.D. and Virginia Hopkins. *What your doctor may not tell you about breast cancer*. New York, Warner Books inc. 2002.

Levine, Peter A., PhD. *Waking the Tiger: Healing Trauma: The Innate Capacity to Transform Overwhelming Experiences.* Berkely, North Atlantic Books, 1997.

Lipton, Bruce H. *The Biology of Belief: Unleashing the Power of Consciousness, Matter, & Miracles.* New York, Hay House, 2009.

Moorjani, Anita. *Dying To Be Me: My Journey from Cancer, to Near Death, to True Healing.* New York, Hay House Inc, 2012.

Moritz. Andreas. *Cancer is Not a Disease. It's a Survival Mechanism. Discover Cancer's Hidden Purpose, Heal its Root Causes, and be Healthier than Ever.* La VergneTN, Lightning Source Inc., 2009.

Nordthrup, Christiane, M.D. *Women's Bodies, Women's Wisdom. Creating Physical and Emotional Health and Healing.* New York, Bantam Dell, 2006.

Overbruggen, Rob van, Ph.D. *Healing Psyche. Patterns and Structure of Complementary Psychological Cancer Treatment (CPCT).* Charleston USA, Book Surge Publishing, 2006.

Siegel, Bernie S, M.D. *Love, Medicine and Miracles: Lessons Learned about Self-Healing from a Surgeon's Experience with Exceptional Patients.* New York, Harper and Row, 1986.

Simonton, Carl, Stephanie-Simonton. *Getting Well Again: The Bestselling Classic About the Simontons' Revolutionary Lifesaving Self-Awareness Techniques.* New York, Bantam Books Inc., 1978.

www.ingramcontent.com/pod-product-compliance
Lightning Source LLC
Chambersburg PA
CBHW051522170526
45165CB00002B/568